Good Living Practices

THE BEST FROM AYURVEDA, YOGA, AND MODERN SCIENCE FOR ACHIEVING OPTIMAL HEALTH, HAPPINESS, AND LONGEVITY

RAMMOHAN RAO, PhD

Good Living Practices

The Best from Ayurveda, Yoga, and Modern Science for Achieving Optimal Health, Happiness, and Longevity

Rammohan Rao, PhD

Published by: KaivalyaWellness.com

ISBN: 978-0-578-67305-9

COPYRIGHT ©2020 BY RAMMOHAN RAO. All rights reserved. No part of this publication may be reproduced, distributed, or transmitted in any form or by any means, including photocopying, recording, or other electronic or mechanical methods, without the prior written permission of the publisher, except in the case of brief quotations embodied in critical reviews and certain other noncommercial uses permitted by copyright law. For further information, please contact the author at **rrao2020kw@gmail.com**

DISCLAIMER: This book serves as an educational guide and is not intended to diagnose, prevent, or treat any disease, nor do the contents advocate replacing standard medical care. The information provided is also not a substitute for professional medical advice. Although the intention is to provide preventive guidelines, it does not replace preventive medical approaches recommended by a qualified healthcare practitioner. While the "Good Health and Wellness Tips" provided at the end of each section have been safely used by many people, as with any health approach, the results cannot be guaranteed due to numerous variables. The author and/or publisher are not responsible for any adverse effects that may result from the natural approaches presented in this book. It is highly recommended that you consult your healthcare provider regarding procedures in this book before making any changes to your current medical treatment.

PRAISE FOR GOOD LIVING PRACTICES

"With years of research and clinical experience, Dr. Ram Rao shares details of his understanding of the healing journey for chronic disease in his book, Good Living Practices*. He uses a unique approach, combining Western science and the Eastern science of Ayurveda and Yoga. This is a great gift for all those looking for alternative healing and willing to take responsibility for their health and healing."*

Dr. William M. Dean, MD (Urology), AD (Doctor of Ayurveda), author of *Foods Heal: Why Certain Foods Help You Feel Your Best* and *The IC Bladder Pain Syndrome: The Alternative Medical Treatment for Interstitial Cystitis.*

"Good Living Practices *is a comprehensive book describing a holistic approach to living, with an extraordinarily good understanding of physical, mental, and emotional health and their correlation. Following the simple tips and practices elaborated in the book will benefit one and all."*

Prof. Yogesh Desai, PhD, Department of Civil Engineering, Indian Institute of Technology, Bombay

"Dr. Ram Rao is one of very few scientists who can legitimately advise us on how best to live well, full of vitality and joy. In Good Living Practices*, he eloquently and succinctly outlines how many of the ancient Eastern wellness practices are now backed by cutting edge science, which can and should help us design and prioritize our lifestyle and practices. This is a must-read for anyone looking for more than what our Western medical approach and daily experience have to offer."*

Dr. Dave Jenkins, MBChB, Founder and Director-SurfAid

*"*Good Living Practices *is an excellent template for a health-conscious lifestyle that helps you enjoy life to its fullest potential. It is a perfect blend of science and ancient Vedic wisdom."*

Dr. Suhas Kshirsagar, BAMS, MD (Ayurveda), Director, Ayurvedic Healing Inc. Best selling author of *The Hot Belly Diet* and *Change Your Schedule, Change Your Life*

"Dr. Ram Rao was passionately involved in experimental biology for more than thirty years. He has also spent more than fifteen years trying to understand the Indian system of healing practices, including Ayurveda, Yoga, meditation, and herbs used for medical reasons. His book, Good Living Practices, *shares his discoveries and explains how these tools and techniques work. This is a book worth reading closely."*

Dr. Yogish Kudva, Professor of Medicine,
Consultant-Division of Endocrinology, Mayo Clinic, Rochester, MN

"Finally, a health book that deeply resonates "true" to every cell in your body. A common-sense book filled with uncommon wisdom, each page drips with practical pearls for mind-body-emotions, of a depth, dimension, and veracity that you have likely never heard, or felt, before. Looking for a book that transcends today's morass of conflicting advice and endless parade of fanatic fad diets? Look no further. Good Living Practices *will make you hungry for the healthy way of life it espouses—dig in!"*

Dr. Nancy Lonsdorf, MD, award-winning Integrative Ayurvedic physician, speaker, and author of *The Healthy Brain Solution for Women Over Forty - 7 Keys to Staying Sharp, On or Off Hormones* and *A Woman's Best Medicine: Health, Happiness and Long Life through Maharishi Ayurveda*

"The book is a unique blend of Ayurveda, Yoga, and modern evidence-based science, and is written in an engaging style that is easily understood by those who are not familiar with the Eastern sciences or medical research. Dr. Rammohan

Rao utilizes his background as a neuroscientist, yoga instructor, and Ayurvedic Practitioner to describe a variety of healthy habits that the reader can choose from to incorporate into their daily living. This book is a great blueprint for establishing healthy habits based on physical, mental, and emotional health and is a very enjoyable read!"

Dr. Diana I. Lurie, PhD. Professor of Neuropharmacology, The University of Montana; Chair, National Ayurveda Medical Association-Certification Board

"Full of interesting case stories and handy self-care tips, Good Living Practices *brings together ancient wisdom and cutting-edge science, inspiring readers to experience greater health and vibrancy of body, mind, and emotions. This book will be helpful for all who wish to enjoy life to the full."*

Dr. Alakananda Ma, MBBS (UK), AD (Doctor of Ayurveda)
Founder & Director, Alandi Ayurveda Gurukula

"In this user-friendly and highly practical book, Dr. Rammohan Rao illuminates how ancient yogic and ayurvedic wisdom may be applied to our modern lives to achieve optimal health and happiness. He shares compelling scientific studies, as well as vignettes from his own life and the life of his clients, to demonstrate that longevity and fulfillment arise from attention to all dimensions of our human experience: physical, mental, and emotional. He provides clear and manageable steps for tuning the body, sculpting the mind, and transforming emotional turmoil into a calm, compassionate embrace of our essential goodness. By implementing the simple but profound practices suggested by Dr. Rao, you will embark on a unique journey of healing and growth."

Dr. Sudha Prathikanti, MD, Clinical Professor of Psychiatry, School of Medicine, University of California, San Francisco

"In the world of modern yoga, we forget all too often that traditional practice is more than just asana. With Good Living Practices, *Dr. Rao reminds us that a well-rounded, truly transformative training includes not only a physical discipline, but proper diet, a positive life outlook, meditation, and, most importantly, selfless service to all humanity. GLP is an excellent instructional manual for every Yoga student, no matter their experience or school of choice."*

Richard Rosen, yoga instructor; Author of *Original Yoga: Rediscovering the Traditional Practices of Yoga, Pranayama: Beyond the Fundamentals, Yoga for 50+,* and *The Yoga of Breath*

"Ram is uniquely qualified to share the wisdom found within the pages of Good Living Practices. *In his own life, he fully integrates a curious spirit and scientific training with a sincere pursuit of Yoga and Ayurveda. This synthesis provides a book all of us have been waiting for: a grounded, easy-to-read owners' manual that combines the best of modern scientific knowledge with a contemporary understanding of Vedic wisdom. Health includes all aspects of who we are, and Dr. Rao acknowledges this with good physical, mental, and emotional practices. We need all of these to enjoy wellness. I highly recommend everyone read this book and implement these sound, evidence-based tips and techniques for good living."*

Felicia Tomasko, RN, C-IAYT, CAP, Editor-in-Chief, LA YOGA Magazine. President, Bliss Network

BONUSES

BOOST YOUR IMMUNE SYSTEM

Having a strong immune system helps to ward off all kinds of infections. Stay healthy with these immunity-boosting recipes to ward off colds, coughs, and all types of infections.

SHARPEN AND KEEP YOUR MEMORY

While memory lapses occur as we age, a rapid decline in memory loss may be a pathological condition. Thanks to intensive research efforts, there are steps you can take to protect and sharpen your mind. This report explains some of the most effective proactive tips you can take to counteract memory losses and cognitive decline.

MAKING MEDITATION SIMPLE

Take a deep breath and relax. Adopt meditation as a habit and it becomes a most simple and powerful technique with huge benefits including peace of mind, anti-aging, less stress, and more experiences of happiness. Whether you are just getting started with meditation or are a seasoned practitioner you will find the tips in this report easier and more accessible.

DOWNLOAD THESE FREE REPORTS AT:

www.KaivalyaWellness.com

FOREWORD

DR. BAXTER BELL, MD
C-IAYT

&

DR. DALE BREDESEN, MD

This book could not have come at a better time. For those living in the US, there is a healthcare cost and access crisis that is being poorly addressed. And at the same time, the World Health Organization (WHO) points out that the vast majority of healthcare dollars in the US are spent on treating conditions that are rooted in poor lifestyle choices. These are familiar conditions we have all heard of: Type 2 diabetes, high blood pressure, heart disease, osteoporosis, obesity, stroke, and some cancers. And the WHO also states clearly that diet and lifestyle choices could dramatically address many of these conditions—preventing 80 percent of heart disease, stroke, type 2 diabetes, and 40 percent of cancers!

One of those lifestyle choices that I personally discovered was Yoga. During a busy, stressful career as a family doctor in the US Midwest, I found myself practicing Yoga for the first time and discovered that it was not only helpful for my physical body but maybe more importantly helpful for my mental-emotional well-being as well. I was hooked!

Fast forward a dozen years, and the benefits of Yoga were so compelling to me that I had left my busy family practice, moved to California, completed training as a yoga teacher and medical acupuncturist, and started to teach and share what I felt were Yoga's great potentials: a healthier body, a calmer mind and emotions, and a clearer connection to soulful living. It was during this time that I was fortunate to meet Ram Rao while offering classes at the research center where he worked. It was clear to me immediately that Ram had a practiced familiarity with Yoga, its postures, and its breath/meditation practices. In the ensuing years, I would also learn about his contributions to the scientific knowledge on aging and disease, and he would go on to write many informative blog posts as a contributing writer for the blog I co-founded primarily around Yoga and the brain as it ages.

It was during those years that Ram not only completed training as an Ayurvedic Practitioner but went on to become a lead instructor at the Ayurvedic school where he had trained. Around the same time, I was becoming familiar with the underlying tenants of this sister science to Yoga and found that Ayurveda's focus on healthy dietary principles and accessible lifestyle practice complemented and elevated Yoga to a more holistic level than it could achieve on its own.

So, it was with great delight that I was introduced to Ram's new book *Good Living Practices*, which brings these sisters of Ayurveda and Yoga together, plus so much more! This book will provide you with invaluable, accessible tools to achieve the ultimate benefit Ram so clearly articulates in the opening chapter: bringing your body, emotions, and mind into sync—and harvesting the benefits of well-being and optimal health. In addition to these practical methods, Ram backs it all up with some of the most up-to-date science we have on how and why these time-tested tools are so effective for your health and happiness. Enjoy the journey and benefits of adding these practices into your life!

Dr. Baxter Bell, MD
C-IAYT (certified Yoga therapist)

For all of us living in the twenty-first century, chronic illness and ill health are an increasing concern. From Alzheimer's disease to metabolic syndrome to cancer to cardiovascular disease, chronic diseases limit the health spans of nearly all of us. Furthermore, most of these illnesses have proven very difficult to treat with standard, single pharmaceuticals. Fortunately, preventive programs that include nutrition and lifestyle optimization are proving to be very effective for maximizing health span. Indeed, such approaches have been used successfully for type 2 diabetes, hypertension, arthritis, multiple sclerosis, depression, and cognitive decline, among others. Therefore, understanding and utilizing these preventive approaches is critical to establishing and maintaining good health and preventing chronic illness.

Good Living Practices has been written by an author who is uniquely qualified to help us understand and apply the principles of nutrition and lifestyle that have the most beneficial effects on health span; Dr. Rammohan Rao is a highly trained molecular neuroscientist with dozens of publications in peer-reviewed scientific and medical journals, and he combines his scientific knowledge with his experience as an Ayurvedic practitioner, along with his third area of expertise as a yoga instructor. As if these three synergistic areas of expertise were not enough, he also successfully practices these principles in his own life.

Dr. Rao's career has been characterized by repeated success: his scientific research has contributed importantly to the understanding of the fundamental mechanism by which ApoE4, the most common genetic risk factor for Alzheimer's disease, leads to cognitive decline—as well as to the mechanism by which damaged proteins destroy brain cells. He has been highly successful in translating his research findings and clinical experience into successful practices for an optimal health span.

Dr. Rao's success, culminating in his new book, *Good Living Practices*, could not be more timely: for the first time, the average lifespan has begun to decrease, largely due to obesity and chronic illnesses such as type 2 diabetes. We have witnessed the repeated failure of candidate drugs for Alzheimer's disease and other neurodegenerative diseases, thus emphasizing the need for effective preventive strategies. Simultaneously, numerous studies have shown promise with dietary approaches such as the Mediterranean diet, lifestyle approaches such as exercise, sleep, stress management, and brain training, and programs that include combinations of these preventive strategies. But what is the best approach, and why? This is where Dr. Rao's unique qualifications are so critical: he not only can describe the most effective principles and practices, but he can also explain the underlying mechanisms of action.

In our quest for optimal health and longevity, we would all do well to read and practice the excellent living principles described by Dr. Rao. As noted by Joyce Meyer, "The greatest gift you can give your family and the world is a healthy you."

Dr. Dale Bredesen, MD
Founding President, Buck Institute; Professor of Neurology, UCLA; Author of the best selling book, The End of Alzheimer's

THIS BOOK IS DEDICATED TO:

My Grandfather, Pandit Subbaramiah Sarma, who introduced me to good living practices when I was in middle school.

My father, Dr. A.V. Rao, who ensured that I sustain these practices.

My mother, Rajalaxmi Rao, who nurtured and distilled me into what I am today.

My two older siblings Prasad Rao and Dr. Prakash Rao, who always encouraged me to go above and beyond at home, studies, and at work.

My wife, Padma Rao, for her constant support and guidance, for encouraging me to execute my thoughts and ideas into this book, and for all the lively discussions about the good practices.

TABLE OF CONTENTS

INTRODUCTION

Every day, hundreds of thousands of dollars are spent on books, courses, and products for health and wellness, diet and exercise, meal plans, meditation, and information about how to live an emotionally fulfilling and balanced life. Clearly, most of us want to live healthier, happier, and longer lives. So, the question is why, as a society, aren't we achieving these goals?

Here is the biggest problem: Almost all so-called health and wellness programs are incomplete, missing vital components.

Books about diets tend to emphasize food alone, although some do couple eating with exercise. Meanwhile, programs about physical exercise usually focus on the benefits and techniques of particular activities, without describing what to eat or how to address our emotional status. Similarly, advice for our emotions provides tips and interventions, but they do not typically integrate physical practices.

Disease, poor health, and suffering primarily arise when the emotions, mind, and body are out of alignment and function independently of one other. In other words, if you only focus on your body—and pay little attention to your mind or emotions—you invite ill health and suffering into your life.

For instance, let's say you read a book that teaches you how to maintain a quality diet. If you read the book and followed it, you may have done an excellent job of improving your health status (weight, blood pressures, cholesterol, etc.). However, if you continue exploding with emotional outbursts at work and home—and find yourself plopping down in front of the television every night with little to no physical activity—you have only addressed a fraction of yourself.

Or, maybe you have immersed yourself in mindfulness practices through daily meditation and treating others with loving-kindness. While your stress levels will decrease, your compassion for others will rise, and your relationships will improve, what is happening to your physical body and mind? No matter how much emotional work you do, if you continue to eat an imbalanced diet, ignore other aspects of mental health, and live a sedentary lifestyle, you may find your emotional state constantly disrupted by sickness, lethargy, weight gain, and an increasingly fuzzy memory and cognitive state.

You're not alone. Many people tend to focus on only one aspect of their development without understanding why they cannot experience complete fulfillment in their lives. In fact, many people all over the world live in this disharmonious manner, not realizing that their fractionated approach is the main culprit.

Fortunately, there is a better way.

When you work to achieve oneness of the body, mind, and emotions, you will put an end to the vicious cycle of improving only one area of your life to the detriment of the others. With an integrative approach, you will set yourself on a course toward a long, healthy, happy, purposeful, and extraordinary life.

This book emphasizes the importance of keeping the body, mind, and emotions in sync, functioning as one unit. With the right set of tools, you can engage your emotions, mind, and physical body simultaneously to achieve optimal health and wellness throughout your lifetime.

By sharing this unique message, I hope to touch, heal, and inspire you. While this approach may appear low-key at first, please trust that the consistent application of the tools will lead to a powerful, transformational impact in your life. The concepts described in this book are not pulled from the etheric space, but instead are drawn from the very best of Yoga and Ayurveda. They are also amply supported by evidence-based research studies, combined with the wisdom I gained from being a neuroscientist, yoga instructor, and Ayurveda practitioner.

I believe this book will address many common problems people face in our society when seeking a healthy lifestyle. It is my sincere hope that the solutions and sage advice provided in these pages will assist you on your journey to leading a healthy, happy, and harmonious life.

How This Book Began: The Origins of Good Living Practices

I was born into a progressive, well-educated, middle-class family in India as the youngest of three siblings. Throughout childhood, my paternal grandfather regularly visited us, and it was he who taught me about harmonious living. He drew most of his wisdom from Vedic texts,[1] as well as the science of Yoga and Ayurveda. My grandfather is also the one who emphasized the importance of the body-mind-emotions nexus, believing alignment among these entities was critical for living a quality life.

Meanwhile, my father, a chemical engineer and researcher, instilled in us the curiosity trait—leading me to constantly question and investigate the world around me. This trait remained with me throughout college, graduate school, and at the Christian Medical College and Hospital (a leading institution in India), where I pursued a PhD in neurosciences. Always the curious student, my final research project focused on the role of certain brain-resident proteins in sleep apnea, and the effects of toxic chemicals and pesticides on these proteins. These studies paved the way for my future work in the science field, as well as an incredible shift in my understanding of human health and wellness.

Working as a Scientist

After graduation and as I embarked upon a career as a scientist at the world-famous Mayo Clinic in Rochester, Minnesota, I continued to focus on the same set of brain-resident proteins from my earlier research. However, I now wanted to better understand the role of these proteins in brain development and the memory loss associated with Alzheimer's disease. While the research projects were interesting, they ultimately resulted in a reductionist approach, where we attempted to view brain function, human behavior, and emotions as a narrow, finite set of biological changes that take place in a test tube or culture dish.

Frustrated with the research projects—as well as the harsh weather conditions of Minnesota—I decided to move to Northern California to join a newly established aging research institute just outside of San Francisco. The founding director of the Buck Institute for Research on Aging was Dr. Dale Bredesen, a well-known neurologist. Dr. Bredesen provided me with the freedom to explore any aspect of aging and age-associated chronic conditions that affected the brain. I focused on mechanisms that underlie the memory loss associated with Alzheimer's disease. After more than a decade of intense research, we identified novel biochemical pathways and key players that trigger memory loss.

This discovery fetched us fame and recognition, numerous publications in leading peer-reviewed journals, and research funds. Unfortunately, we were still nowhere close to finding the miracle drug to halt, reverse, or delay this dreaded disease. Adding to that frustration was the knowledge that, over the past 15 years, there have been about 200 failed attempts at developing Alzheimer's drugs, at an aggregate cost of billions of dollars. This has led many experts (including me) to question whether the drug-discovery approach for Alzheimer's disease is an optimal one.

In community lectures and talks that I used to deliver, the audience asked a simple question: "Do you have the miracle drug to reverse or stop Alzheimer's disease?" Sadly, I had to reply in the negative.

A Fresh Perspective

During this time, it dawned on me that the modern scientific approach to drug discovery for any health condition is flawed. When scientists design a drug, it is important to understand that what is considered "human" includes not just the physical body and associated symptoms but also the mind and emotions. The human body (together with the mind and emotions) is a highly complex system, composed of cells, tissues, organs, blood vessels, nerves, channels, hormones, chemicals, thoughts, emotions, etc. All of these components are tightly linked and work in tandem.

However, trying to correct a complex functional pathway with a single drug sets the stage for a future, large-scale collapse seen in all of the failed clinical trials. This is why I believe the scientific community continues to hit a wall in its research and development of an effective drug for Alzheimer's disease or other health-related conditions. Instead, the emotions, mind, and body need to be taken into consideration as a whole for any physical, mental, or psychological condition to improve. Sadly, researchers and clinicians have largely ignored this integrative approach.

Despite my frustrations with the non-integrative approaches to treating disease, I only appreciated and understood the true importance of the body-mind-emotions nexus for overall health and wellness when my wife, Padma, suffered from a complex autoimmune condition. Whether it was Alzheimer's disease research, autoimmune conditions, or other health-related issues, I began to realize that a holistic approach was not merely desired but critical.

Eastern Medical Sciences

In my wife's case, the Western medications that she took for her autoimmune condition triggered a host of negative side effects. So, as an ardent believer in the Eastern medicinal system called Ayurveda (with roots in the Vedic texts from approximately 5000 BCE), Padma sought Ayurvedic treatment for her health issue. Back in the early 2000s, there was only one Ayurveda institution near Sacramento, Grass Valley, which offered people both teaching and treatment. We both agreed it was worth a shot.

Padma and I showed up in this small, sleepy town and met with an Ayurveda practitioner. At the end of a thorough three-hour consult, the practitioner provided us with a comprehensive to-do list of interventions. I was intrigued by this list. The practitioner's recommendations for the body, mind, and emotions—even though her only "complaint" was based on a *physical* condition—was unheard of and not recommended in the mainstream Western medicinal system.

Despite my reservations, Padma followed the interventions closely. In addition to diet, herbs, physical exercise, and sleep routines, the treatment program also included mental exercise, breath practice, meditation, selfless service, and practicing loving-kindness. In just six months, Padma experienced a dramatic improvement in her health. In fact, she was entirely symptom-free!

During one of our follow-up meetings with the same practitioner, I also met with Dr. Halpern, the Director of the California College of Ayurveda, who asked if I might be interested in pursuing and teaching Ayurveda. Looking back, I assumed he most likely believed that my neuroscience background could benefit the students of Ayurveda. Despite my full-time laboratory research, I enrolled in the forty-two month Ayurveda program. This was also the time that Padma and I became serious students of Yoga.

My wife remained symptom-free, and I continued my studies to become a certified Ayurveda practitioner, a faculty teacher at the California College of Ayurveda, and a 200-hour Registered Yoga Teacher from Yoga Alliance. As I delved deeper into these sciences, I soon discovered the true meaning of several concepts regarding the body-mind-emotions nexus that my grandfather taught me so many years ago. Ayurveda and Yoga are part of the complex Vedic texts, with Ayurveda focusing on good health, wellness, and healing—while Yoga describes the behavioral, emotional, and spiritual aspects of living.

Yoga empowers us by advocating a unique, personalized lifestyle practice, through physical and mental exercises, meditation, positive thoughts, and selfless service. All of this is intending to improve one's physical, mental, and emotional health. Meanwhile, Ayurveda relies on a comprehensive, personalized therapeutic program that includes diet, sleep, an affirmative disposition, and physical and mental exercise to promote an extraordinary life.

The practices of Yoga and Ayurveda are meant to bring clarity to the emotions, calm the mind, and strengthen the body, thereby developing a deeper emotional-mind-body awareness. Thus, a complete, personalized program drawn from these Eastern medicinal sciences and supported by evidence-based research studies not only ensures that the body, mind, and emotions are in equanimity, but this practice also serves as a basis for harmonious living. This has been evident in the health status of the majority of patients that have sought Ayurvedic treatment from me. I have put them all in some form of comprehensive body-mind-emotions program, and most who followed the program judiciously noticed a remarkable improvement in their health. These positive results have become the inspiration for this book.

Good Living Practices, Defined

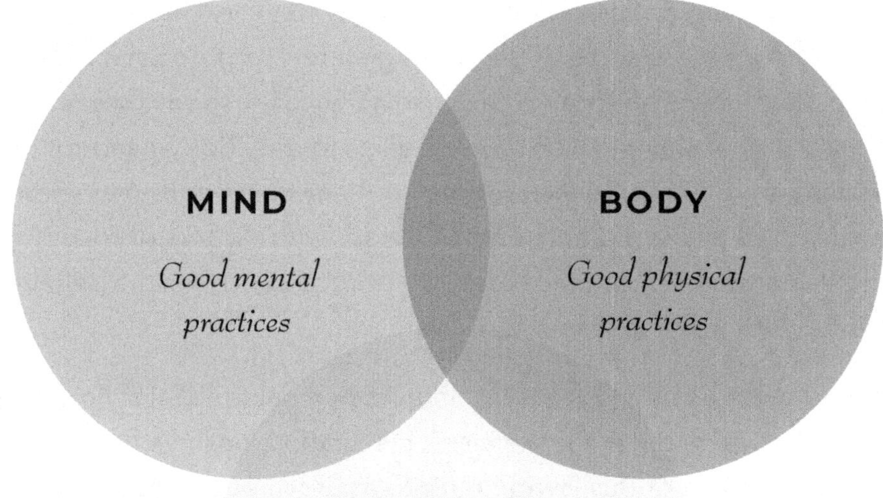

FIGURE 1: GOOD LIVING PRACTICES

Good Living Practices (GLP) include Good Physical Practices (Body), Good Mental Practices (Mind), and Good Emotional Practices (Emotions). GLP includes tools that keep these three aspects (body, mind, and emotions) in sync for optimal health and living. Pay attention to the "Tips on Good Living Practices" provided at the end of each chapter to keep the body, mind, and emotions in sync. For best results, engage in these practices daily, 24/7.

In keeping with these ancient philosophies, I have developed the Good Living Practices toolkit. Throughout this book, I offer a definitive resource on how to use these tools to foster physical, mental, and emotional health.

As I have been alluding to, each of us has three different facets that we consider "human," including: (1) a physical body, (2) a mental body, and (3) an emotional body (Figure 1). While these three facets appear as independent entities, such a limiting belief is the root cause of suffering and disease. Instead, if we believe that we are a combination of body, mind, and emotions, and act accordingly, it is possible to lead a harmonious life with significantly increased protection from illness and disease.

Good Living Practices (GLP), then, are the tools that keep these three entities (body, mind, and emotions) in sync. For optimal health and living, GLP should be practiced daily, 24/7.

What You Will Learn

At the physical level, the first set of practices (*Good Physical Practices*) promotes harmonious living through good eating practice, physical exercises, and tuning the body. Those of us who incorporate Good Physical Practices into our daily routine find ourselves feeling empowered and positive about our direction in life. In addition, Good Physical Practices help us to gain strength and immunity, to feel energetic, and to find life enjoyable through mindful eating, physical exercise, and "tuning" the body to nurture one's physical senses.

At the level of the mind, GLP includes *Good Mental Practices,* which is about reinforcing the structural and functional aspects of the brain. This can be achieved through sleeping well, mental training exercises, and engaging in selfless service. Incorporating these practices into your life will lower the risk of serious health problems, reduce stress and improve mood, enhance mental clarity, and help you to make wise decisions.

Finally, at the level of the emotions, GLP includes Good Emotional Practices, which help to attain wisdom and cultivate harmonious thoughts that, in turn, reduce mental conflict and promote a fully functional life. Good Emotional Practices involve using suitable tools to perceive, understand, control, evaluate, and express emotions. This enables us to be aware of life's daily dramas, control emotional upheavals, and act effortlessly to experience complete peace and joy. The tools that encompass Good Emotional Practices include meditation, the cultivation of a defined set of five positive emotions (known as the "noble five"), and overcoming emotional deterrents.

As you read through this book, I strongly recommend that you pay attention to the "Tips on Good Living Practices" provided at the end of each chapter to keep the body, mind, and emotions in sync. It is important to apply these tools daily in your life to detoxify the body, retrain the mind, and purify the emotions. While there are numerous ideas provided in these tips, I suggest you start with just a few at first to prevent feeling overwhelmed. Then, over time, you can incorporate more tips into your routine as you see fit since the more tools you use, the more transformational your results will be. You will also find it helpful when choosing which tools to use to combine strategies from each of the three sections of this book to ensure a fully integrated approach of body, mind, and emotions. Now, I invite you to join me on this journey that will nurture your mind, body, and emotions in a way that will lead you to happiness, satisfaction, clarity, pure joy, and bliss.

PART I

GOOD PHYSICAL PRACTICES

The first of the Good Living Practices (Good Physical Practices) allows you to achieve high levels of empowerment and positivity. When you incorporate these principles into your routine, you'll feel more optimistic about your life choices, improve your energy, and strengthen your body, mind, and emotions—all while increasing your overall enjoyment of life.

GOOD PHYSICAL PRACTICES INCLUDE:

CHAPTER 1: EATING MINDFULLY.

This chapter features healthy eating practices that will help you understand that we are *what, when, how, why,* and *where* we eat.

CHAPTER 2: THE AEROBIC BODY

A daily physical exercise regimen is the secret to remaining physically strong and active. This chapter will highlight the benefits of exercises as well as the effects on your well-being when you *don't* make exercise part of your life.

CHAPTER 3: TUNING THE BODY

You take your vehicle for maintenance to avoid problems while driving—so why not do the same with your body? In this chapter, I will discuss the rationale for tuning the body through periodic detoxification techniques that anyone can do from the comfort of home.

If you incorporate the practices from Chapters 1-3 into your life, you will find them to be extremely helpful for warding off most physical illnesses. You'll also enjoy the additional benefits these practices contribute to the overall health of your mind and emotions, allowing you to live your life to the fullest.[2]

CHAPTER 1

EATING MINDFULLY

"By eating pure food, the mind becomes pure"

CHHANDOGYA UPANISHAD, 7.26.2

"Tell me what you eat, and I will tell you what you are," declared French gastronome Jean Anthelme Brillat-Savarin. Similarly, the well-known German philosopher and anthropologist Ludwig Feuerbach reminds us, "You are what you eat." While both men may not have meant that their quotations be taken literally, what we eat truly plays a vital role in our quality of life.

Vedic texts, Ayurveda, and Yoga philosophy also support the concept of eating consciously. These texts explain that if digestion is not optimal, it can destabilize the emotions, mind, and body, creating imbalances in each. Most of us routinely experience digestive disturbances, and whether it's acute or chronic, indigestion can cause discomfort and/or embarrassment. Because the gut serves as the entry point to our complete physiological system, optimal functioning is vital to prevent imbalances not only in the body but also with the mind and emotions. By correcting imbalances, proper digestion brings a swift end to suffering while also preventing future disease and promoting a long, healthy, and high-quality life.

In addition to conscious eating to promote optimal digestion, the Vedic texts also stress the importance of being in tune with nature while eating mindfully. Food connects us with nature and allows us to become one with it. When we live in harmony with nature, we experience peace of mind and a well-balanced emotional state. In contrast, when we are out of harmony with nature, we experience poor health and suffering.[3]

At this point, you may be asking, "So, how do I improve my diet, digestion, and connection to nature, and thereby ward off disease while improving my physical, mental, and emotional state?" The easiest way to begin is to break mindful eating into the *what, when, how, where,* and *why* you eat, which I will describe in more detail below.

You Are WHAT You Eat

For anyone seeking specific dietary recommendations, there are hundreds of books and manuals on the market that bombard us with mixed messages about diet and nutrition, and those messages have changed dramatically over time. Initially, fats were enemy numero uno, so everyone loaded up on carbs. That is, until carbs got a raw deal, thanks to Robert Atkins, and fats returned to the dining plate. Eventually, we were told all carbs are not created equal, so with the concept of good versus bad carbs, certain "acceptable" carbs returned to the table. Then, protein-rich and Paleo diets staked their claims in the food contest as well. Meanwhile, the raw eaters fought for the top rung in the gastronome chain, along with vegetarians and vegans. Recently, we've seen a steady stream of foodists claiming the benefits of fasting or ketogenic diets.

It's no surprise, then, that what we should or shouldn't eat has turned into a burning quagmire. In this book, I will refrain from recommending a specific diet; instead, I will emphasize what not to eat and provide examples of better food choices.

PAY ATTENTION TO PRANA

According to the Vedic texts, foods need to be high in "prana," which I define as the vital or singular force that keeps the body, mind, and emotions integrated into a single, unified entity. Experiencing a "high prana" state is an effortless experience where the ego falls away, time vanishes, and our body, mind, and emotions unite as a whole. The moment becomes intrinsically blissful and rewarding. Initially, it requires great effort to access this state of being. And while it does not sustain for long, the experience is extremely powerful.

Whether you realize it or not, you have experienced moments of the "highest prana" at some point in time. Think back to moments of pure bliss in your life. Maybe you felt it when holding your newborn child for the first time. Or maybe engaging in selfless service induces that high prana state. For others, something as simple as stepping outside in the early morning hours allows one to access this bliss.

When it comes to eating, you need to experience a similar state of high prana and that feeling comes only when you eat prana-rich foods. The rule of thumb to determine if a food has high or low-quality prana is to consider its source. In other words, the closer the food is to its own natural state, the higher the prana. The farther the food is from its original state, the less prana it possesses. Thus, foods that are handled by multiple people or that are manipulated through various devices have low prana. In Table 1 (below), I provide a list of foods that are low, medium, and high in prana that you can use to evaluate your diet and make suitable changes or modifications.

LOW PRANA	MEDIUM PRANA	HIGH PRANA
Commercial dairy milk and milk products	Commercially available non-dairy milk and milk products	Fresh, unadulterated dairy milk and milk products
Red meat	Vegetables not in season	Freshly prepared non-dairy milk
Refrigerated packaged foods	Fruits not in season	Vegetables in season
Food prepared and left in the fridge for >24 hours and reheated	Microwavable ready-to-eat foods	Fruits in season

LOW PRANA	MEDIUM PRANA	HIGH PRANA
Prepared food that has gone through several rounds of refrigeration and reheating	Deep-fried vegetables	Naturally ripened fruits
Deep-fried, meat-based foods	Food prepared, left in the fridge for less than 24 hours and reheated	Freshly prepared foods
Cold, bulk prepared beverages	Unbleached flour	Warm-hot food
Beverages containing artificial ingredients		Natural sugars
Canned drinks		Freshly baked foods
Canned fruits		Fresh shallow fried foods
Canned vegetables		Steamed or sautéed vegetables
Canned foods		Freshly prepared beverage
Vegan meat and other meat substitutes		Whole grain or coarse grain flour
Highly milled, bleached flour		

While there are immense benefits to the body, mind, and emotions from consuming high-prana foods, low-medium prana foods will prevent you from sustaining optimal health.

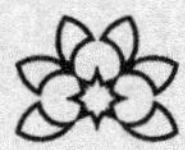

CASE STUDY

Martin was a busy lawyer who lived alone and had little time to cook, much less focus on where his food came from. His typical schedule included a large latte from the local coffee shop near his firm. He rarely ate anything for breakfast since he was typically rushing into the office for a meeting.

After client meetings and court appearances, he would return to his desk to catch up on email and have fast food delivered to eat as he worked. By seven or eight, he was too exhausted to go to the grocery store, so he would meet up with some colleagues for a few drinks and appetizers. Within a few hours, Martin would return to his apartment and fall asleep watching the late-night shows.

Although he was young and fit, within a few years of this routine, his health suffered. He put on some weight, and in the mornings, he felt foggy and forgetful. By mid-afternoon, he wanted nothing more than to take a nap. And at night, he would toss and turn, taking antacids for the acid reflux that was becoming more and more irritating.

Clearly, Martin's diet consists of almost all low-prana foods. From the morning rush of caffeine, to the fast-food midday, and the evening habit of drinking and eating close to bedtime, this was a recipe for disaster. Fortunately, Martin took charge and made some significant changes.

When a friend suggested that Martin pay closer attention to his diet, he began to focus on changing his ways. He started slowly, at first just eliminating the coffee and substituting it with a cup of tea and a piece of fruit. For lunch, he still ordered out, but he substituted the burgers and fries with fresh salads and warm soups. He coordinated food delivery from the local grocery store in his city, and he found a few simple recipes that took little time to prepare for dinner. By returning home right after work, he had a few hours to relax and allow his food to digest before going to bed.

While he would still meet his colleagues for the occasional happy hour, this became the exception rather than the rule. Almost immediately, the brain-fog lifted, and he felt much more energetic throughout the day. Over time, the acid reflux symptoms diminished, and today he no longer takes any medication for this condition. He also enjoyed some weight loss, providing him with the energy and motivation to join a running club before work.

Martin's switch to higher-prana foods made all the difference. Remember, foods that have not faced any interference in their habitat and are close to their natural state have the highest prana. Now, take a moment to consider your own diet. Look at Table 1 (above) and determine if you are, like Martin, eating low-prana foods or if your diet consists of high-prana choices.

Now, let's get into the specifics of low and high-prana foods in the categories of dairy, non-dairy, meat, and produce:

DAIRY

When I was young and growing up in India, the cattleman would bring the cows or water buffaloes to an area close to his customers. The cattle were fed a mixture of grains and grass, and the cattleman would manually milk them and distribute the raw milk to the customers. Since we did not own a refrigerator, we consumed the milk on the same day.

The cattle lived in an open, fresh atmosphere and ate natural food. They were not subjected to any milking devices, there were no injections, and the cattleman performed the milking operation with respect and love. For us, pasteurization was akin to heating the milk on a stove until a thin layer of cream formed on the surface. That was as far as our milk was "processed."

This pure, unadulterated milk possessed high prana. Because we consumed it on the same day, the life energy lived in that milk in its purest form. Compared to today's world, there is a stark difference. Even though the dairy industry is working to adopt good practices, including optimal animal health and welfare, proper feeding and water, and ensuring good milking hygiene and environment, modern-day milk has very low prana.

Huge batches of milk from the animals pass through various grids as they get mixed, pasteurized, homogenized, and packaged. The final end product is milk that needs to be refrigerated for it to last several days. Through this process, the milk enters an extremely low-prana state. Today, the more we witness exponential growth in the number of people complaining of dairy/lactose intolerance, it's really no surprise, considering the intricate link between low-prana milk and physical imbalance. For this reason, it is extremely important to be mindful of your body's reaction to dairy if you choose to ingest these products.

DAIRY ALTERNATIVES

Health issues are associated with these foods, as well. While dairy is as natural as it comes (when it's straight from the cattle), dairy alternatives are man-made and processed, with comparatively low prana. Although manufacturers attempt to mimic the consistency, taste, viscosity, and the nutritional benefits of dairy, this substitute for the real thing is actually full of synthetic chemicals.

One particularly concerning ingredient in dairy alternatives is carrageenan. Carrageenan is a polysaccharide that's extracted from seaweed and has no nutritional value. Manufacturers add it to soups, ice creams, and dairy to thicken, emulsify, and improve the texture. But did you know that immunologists actually use carrageenan and other polysaccharides to stimulate inflammation in human tissue in a laboratory setting? In fact, when researchers expose laboratory animals to low concentrations of carrageenan, they develop profound inflammation. Meanwhile, companies continue to add this ingredient to our food, leaving the consumer susceptible to the negative health effects.

MEAT

Like some of the dairy and dairy alternatives, the Ayurveda texts consider meat to be low-prana food. While some people justify eating animals as a means of improving their health, many studies reveal that animal products actually do more harm than good.

Both the World Health Organization (WHO) and The International Agency for Research on Cancer (IARC) have classified processed meat—especially red meat—as a carcinogen.[4] The folks in the meat industry may claim that they treat the cattle humanely and feed them organic food. However, the issue is not about what the cattle eat or graze on, or their living conditions. It is about their state of body and mind just before they are slaughtered.

Animals are not only intelligent and sensitive creatures, but they too suffer and feel pain in the same way that we do. Keeping animals locked in confinement, denying them a natural life, stunning them, or jolting them with an electric current, and finally allowing the animal to bleed out while it is still alive, are both abhorrently cruel practices and highly stressful situations for the animals.[5]

Aquatic creatures, birds, reptiles, and land animals all have similar biochemical, neurochemical, and pain pathways—and the same fight-or-flight responses as humans. Hence, they respond to stressful situations by releasing hormones like adrenaline, cortisol, and other glucocorticoids. These deleterious neurochemicals, stress hormones, and other signaling molecules circulate in the animal's brain and body, wreaking havoc to its physiological system.

This, then, is the low-prana state of our food as we consume that meat dish. Not only that, but numerous research studies demonstrate that any kind of stress in animals compromises the tenderness, perishability, color, and shelf life of the meat. If that isn't bad enough, research studies have tied red meat to an increased risk of diabetes, heart disease, and various cancers, as well as an elevated mortality rate.[6]

PRODUCE

Like humans, birds, and animals, vegetables and fruits also connect closely with the earth, moon, and sun. Between the earth's rotation, tilt, and revolution around the sun, these seasonal changes influence consumable crops. Because a food's prana is specific to its season, knowing which produce to eat during a particular time of year is important. In addition to prana, eating produce that's in season aids digestion and improves health.[7]

While mango, melons, beans, cucumbers, and berries grow during the summer season, squash, sweet potatoes, and pomegranates are winter plants. If you're not sure what and when to buy your produce, pay a visit to your neighborhood farmer's market, since they only carry produce that is fresh and in-season.

Both vegetables and fruits are rich sources of vitamins, minerals, phytonutrients, antioxidants, phytochemicals, healthy sugars, electrolytes, fiber, fat, and protein—all of which have immense health benefits. For fruits, you'll want to determine if the fruit is ripe; as fruits ripen, they become sweeter, softer, and more palatable. In fact, ripening fruits produce several phytochemicals and antioxidants.

Unfortunately, due to the large demand for fruits, growers sometimes resort to poor harvesting practices and pluck them before they ripen. Birds, insects, and molds attack ripe fruits, too, which is another reason farmers don't always allow them to ripen completely. Some growers artificially ripen the fruit by using gases and chemicals, even though they can be harmful to human health.[8] However, some fruits (especially those that belong to the melon family) cannot ripen once they are picked. Not only are unripened and artificially ripened fruits highly acidic (leading to indigestion), but they also have low prana.

Because fruits are moist, nourishing, and rich in sugars, they constitute a meal. Therefore, fruits should be eaten alone, without combining them with other foods. According to Vedic texts, if fruits are combined with a regular meal, their presence reduces a prana-rich meal into a low-prana meal that can affect digestion and metabolism. The science behind this relates to one of the factors that determine the efficiency of the gut function: gastrointestinal transit time (GI transit time).

GI transit time determines how long food remains in the stomach, small intestine, and large intestine. If transit time is too short, the food will pass through the gut so rapidly that the body will not be able to absorb the optimum number of nutrients. In contrast, if transit time is long, food passes through the GI tract much more slowly. This results in (1) excess water reabsorption from the intestine, causing the waste product to become more solid and harder to pass, triggering constipation, inflammation, or infection of the colon wall and other bowel syndromes; (2) the production of ammonia and sulfur compounds, which at high concentrations affect the structure and function of the GI tract; and (3) degradation of fats and non-digestible sugars into byproducts that can affect the heart and pancreas.

Thus, when regular food is combined with fruits, the GI transit time is either too slow or too rapid, thereby affecting digestion, absorption, and assimilation of essential components. If you have an underlying health issue and a daily habit of eating meals together with fruits, this can compound the negative effects on your health. That is why, the next time you plan to reach out to fruit granola or fruit yogurt, I recommend you think about the GI transit time and eat wisely. While fruit granola, mango lassi, yogurt, and other fruit-based foods are delicious, they should be avoided—especially if you have health issues.

Another suggestion to benefit fully from produce (vegetables and fruits) is to consider growing it yourself—if you have the motivation, time, and space for it. Even if your space is tight, container or pot gardening is a viable option, too. DIY gardening (by yourself or with a community) reduces the risk of soil-borne diseases, eliminates weed problems, and gives you more control over moisture, temperature, and sunlight. Plus, it's fun and rewarding.

Produce from your own garden is fresh and higher in nutrients when compared to produce that have traveled many miles to reach your local grocery store. If gardening interests you, check out some books to learn more. In fact, your entire family can participate and join in the fun!

Home gardening also allows you to avoid the use of synthetic chemicals, herbicides, and pesticides in favor of natural fertilizers, thereby making the plants healthier. Growing your own produce also allows you to appreciate nature, results in increased physical activity, and keeps your mind calm and peaceful. In addition to cultivating a healthy practice, gardening allows you to remain more grounded and centered—something you will learn more about in later sections of this book (see Chapter 2: The Aerobic Body and Chapter 7: Meditation).

You can also grow your own produce through Homa farming—a high-quality organic farming practice. In Homa farming, the atmosphere is the most important source of nutrition, so this practice involves purifying and stimulating the air through small, controlled, cleansing fires and the use of animal manure and compost to nourish the soil. According to the Vedic texts, Homa farming not only stimulates timely rains, but it also nourishes the plants and prevents plant disease, naturally. The cleansing fires release nourishing substances into the atmosphere, and when they accumulate to a certain threshold, it triggers precipitation of the moisture in the atmosphere—resulting in rainfall. This is similar to the "cloud seeding" process of adding chemicals to clouds to increase rainfall.

PRANA AND STRESS

Before you eat, it is important to reflect on your own physical, mental, and emotional state, especially as it relates to your stress level. Do you have too much drama in your life? Feeling overwhelmed? Are you experiencing fear, worry, anxiety, anger, rage, depression, or irritability?

Mental and emotional issues trigger the fight-or-flight response—the same response that your body activates when you face dangerous situations. When your body enters a fight-or-flight state, it releases neurochemicals like adrenaline and cortisol, and they can wreak havoc with your digestion. Therefore, it is imperative to remain in a calm state while eating.[9]

If you are feeling high levels of stress, do not eat until you can quiet your body and mind. This same principle holds true for the person who is preparing the food. Calm food preparation and eating allow both the preparer and person consuming the food to remain in a high-prana zone.

My grandfather used to recite mantras when we sat down to eat. Mantras are sacred sounds or utterances that bring peace to the body, mind, and soul. They are pleasant-sounding and harmonious and can have a positive, energetic effect.[10] Even if you are not into mantras, you can listen to the sounds of nature or some soft music to help you feel more calm and stress-free.

You Are WHEN You Eat

Our close connection with nature helps us to become aware of the role of the sun in our digestion. Our digestive system's internal clock is regulated by the circadian rhythms of the body to keep it functioning on a defined schedule. The digestive system clock and circadian rhythms are highly influenced by sunlight. That is why, according to Ayurveda, at noon—when the sun is at its peak in the sky—digestion is at its strongest. Similarly, digestive capacity is at its lowest during dawn or in the evening, when the sun is either rising or setting.

For these reasons, Ayurveda's dietary guidelines recommend that you eat your largest meal midday, with smaller meals in the morning and evening. Timing your meals based on the sun's position prevents weight gain and the onset of other digestive related problems, as well as ensuring harmony in the body.

Also, consider how frequently you eat. If you are accustomed to eating more than two meals a day, try to leave a four-hour gap between meals. Generally, hunger sets in every four to five hours, but the body also gets used to a specific schedule. Following specific meal times helps to sustain optimal health since it gets you in the habit of eating at the same time every day. Personally, I prefer eating a big meal at noon and a small meal as the sun sets, and I ensure that I stick to these timings daily.

Research supports the aforementioned recommendations. Studies reveal that having lunch as the main meal of the day (before 2 p.m.) helped subjects lose an average of twenty-two pounds in twenty weeks. Conversely, studies indicate that late-lunch eaters—as well as people eating their meals at random times—experience greater insulin resistance, a risk factor for diabetes.[11] Healthy eating also relates to the food-sleep connection. First, it is advisable to maintain a three-hour gap between dinner and sleep. According to Ayurveda texts, a light meal coinciding with the setting sun is a healthy practice to keep the body-mind-emotions in a harmonious state. The texts also recommend refraining from any caloric food after the last meal of the day—and to break the fast after a minimum of twelve hours.

Modern research agrees with Ayurveda, as studies indicate that a "fasting window" of twelve to fifteen hours between the last meal at night and the first meal the next morning activates the brain cells, allowing them to switch from glucose to fat metabolism. This leads to the release of fat products that have numerous protective effects on the brain.[12]

So, what could this look like in practice? I aim for seven hours of sleep, with a habit of waking up early, and I tend to finish my last meal of the day around 7:00 p.m., with a 10:00 p.m. bedtime. My goal is to maintain a twelve-to-fifteen-hour fast between dinner and the next day's meal, which means I won't eat again until at least 7:00 a.m.

Please note that prolonged fasting, severely cutting back on calories, or fasting mimetics (drugs that mimic the fasting process, despite food intake) can all negatively impact your health. These practices can lead to mental fog, fatigue, weight gain, weakness, the inability to work long hours, and/or unexplained pain. Unfortunately, scientists and technology leaders have jumped on these dieting fads, promoting the false impression that extreme fasting, drastic calorie reduction, and fasting mimetics are the simplest and cheapest ways to improve health and longevity.

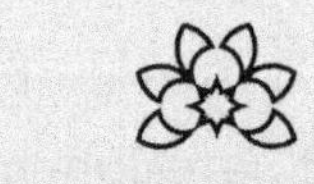

CASE STUDY

Jana works in an office setting, which requires her to sit many hours each day in a cubicle. When she noticed that her weight kept creeping up on the scale, she began paying attention to the office talk of fasts and other fad diets. After talking to a few of her trusted colleagues about the pros and cons of each, Jana decided to embark on a prolonged fasting program. At first, the results were dramatic: She dropped pounds rapidly, allowing her to finally fit back into clothes that had become way too snug.

However, after a few months, the numbers on the scale seemed to freeze. No matter what she did, the weight loss ground to a halt. Not only that, but she was noticing that she was becoming extremely forgetful—especially at work, where having a sharp mind was critical for quality job performance. And when she visited her family doctor for a routine exam, Jana was horrified to learn that her blood work indicated a pre-diabetic condition. "Could it be the fast?" she timidly asked her doctor.

Of course, I am not a doctor, but if I had been one of Jana's colleagues, I would have encouraged her to consider periodic fasting instead, which involves avoiding food for one entire day every month. During your fast, drink only water. No solid foods or caloric liquid beverages are recommended during this time.

Unlike Jana's experiment, a monthly periodic fast is much more gentle to the body over time. In fact, researchers have learned that in both the 12- or 24-hour fast, the body's internal recycling program (known as autophagy) rids the body of all the cellular trash, including subcellular organelles, old cell membranes, worn-out cells, and other cellular debris. This allows the body to free up the energy system,[13] and it serves as a crucial defense mechanism against cancer, infection, and neurodegenerative diseases.

My grandfather encouraged this fasting practice, intuitively understanding the benefits to our health and well-being. In his opinion, fasting made us more intelligent, resilient, and motivated to pursue higher aspects of living. With the science to back it up, now we know why.

You Are HOW You Eat

It all begins when you sit to eat—and the recommendations in this section may be a departure from your normal routine. Ayurveda and Yoga philosophy direct us to sit cross-legged on the floor to begin the eating process. This posture keeps the spine tall while relaxing the hip flexors, which prevents overarching of the upper back or slumping of the lower spine. A poor eating posture can compromise digestion. If you have acid reflux, feel bloated or gassy from a meal, in addition to the food prana, you need to check your eating posture as well.

Sitting down on the floor to eat is a common practice in many traditions (see Figure 2). At first, it may feel awkward to sit cross-legged, but I can attest to the benefits, both for eating and strength. After years of getting up and down from a cross-legged sitting position, I have noticed that my lower body strength is better than that of my peers, who always sit on a chair to eat. As we age, it is more important than ever to strengthen the lower body to maintain stability and balance, and continuous routines like this can definitely help. (Note: If you have tight hip flexors or a tight lower back, it will be helpful to sit on a blanket or two, which will tilt the hips forward and make it easier to sit upright.)

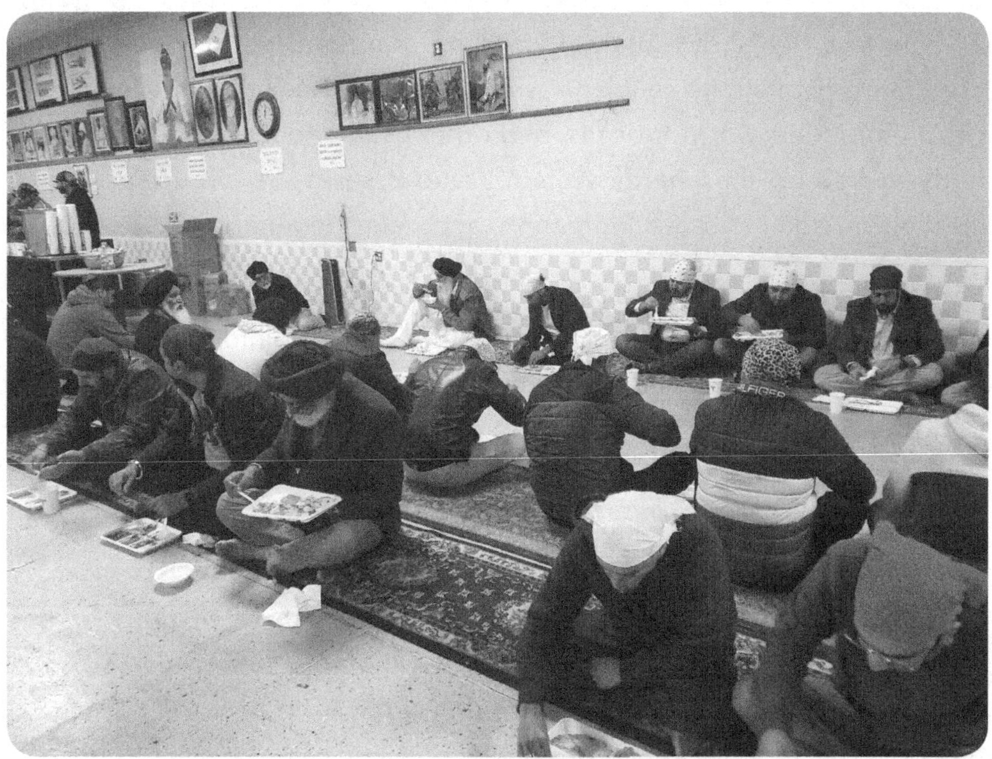

Figure 2: In this image of a free community meal, people are shown sitting on the floor and eating. In many traditions, it's common practice to sit on the floor while eating (as mentioned in the text) as there are many benefits. This picture is of the community dining hall at Gur Nanak Parkash Damdami Taksal-Sikh temple in Tracy, CA.

If you cannot sit on the floor to eat, establish any comfortable sitting position, but make sure that you sit tall and are not overarching or slumping on the seat. Focus your attention on the food, allowing yourself to activate your sense of smell and sight. Absorb the aroma and appreciate the colors, shape, and texture of the various ingredients on the plate.

For those of you who do not say grace or bless the food, you can still evoke pleasurable sensations by giving thanks to all the elements and beings that contributed to the plate of food. You can thank the universe for the sunlight, rain, and the right temperature for the crops to grow. Silently thank the farmer who grew the crops, the animals that helped the farmer, those who brought the raw foods to the market, and finally to the person who cooked the food. This is a simple yet profound way to give thanks.

Giving thanks helps you achieve a state of calm and peace that promotes good digestion. In the Vedic texts, there is one simple mantra to give thanks: "*Annadhata Sukhi Bhava.*" It means, "Let all who provided this food be peaceful." This powerful, heartfelt blessing is an effective form of meditation as well, which I will discuss in greater detail in the next section.

Your food should be fresh and warm. Because it is difficult to appreciate the temperature of the food when you are eating with a fork or a spoon, use your fingers to hold the food and notice if your skin can tolerate the heat. Then, you can either warm up the food further or allow it to cool down to an acceptable temperature. As the seat of acupressure points, your fingers activate nerve endings, so holding your food can lead to a pleasurable sensory experience. It also triggers specific areas in your brain that prepare the mouth and gut for the digestion process.

Now, take a small bite of food and begin chewing. When food enters the mouth, the jaw muscles position the food between the teeth for grinding and crushing. Multiple neural circuits connect the jaw muscles to the brain tissue, and this exchange of information lets your brain determine how much force, momentum, and enzyme activity you need to chew the food.

As you eat the food, aim to chew a minimum of thirty times. This chewing action releases salivary contents that facilitate proper digestion. As chewing continues and the food becomes softer, both the food and the saliva work their way into the esophagus and stomach, where the next step of digestion occurs. When the saliva levels reach a certain threshold in the stomach, this stimulates the satiety centers in the brain. At this point, the brain sends I-feel-full signals to the stomach.

Not only will thorough chewing help you realize that you are full (and therefore eat less food), but research studies show that the more you chew, the more calories you burn during the process.[14] I consider chewing one of the most natural, safe methods to dampen the hunger response and lose fat!

Incidentally, the same regions in your brain that regulate the eating process are also involved in memory, attention, and learning. It's no surprise, then, that researchers have discovered that improper chewing or masticatory dysfunction triggers alterations in the memory centers of the brain, leading to poor spatial learning and memory deficits.[15] In contrast, chewing increases cerebral blood flow and is associated with better cognitive performance, word recall, and working memory.

According to the Vedic texts, the food placed before you required the collective efforts of people, nature, and its elements. Out of respect, you should not play with the food, and you should avoid criticism and complaints. Instead, politely accept the food set before you. If there is something you don't like, eat what you do like, without resorting to unnecessary comments. Your mind and emotions need to be calm and peaceful, and critical comments create a turbulent state. These negative critiques are "thought energies" as well, and that energy can actually disturb the energy flow of everyone involved in the food chain. (Note: For more on thought energy, refer to Section 3, Chapter 9.)

You Are WHERE You Eat

Not in the car, not in front of the TV or laptop, not while texting, not lying down, and certainly not while reclining on the bed. Eating is a sacred activity; it is a metamorphosis that nourishes and sustains you. Therefore, you need to ensure that eating is the sole activity that you are engaging in, and this should not be accompanied by other tasks.

Eating should not take place in a loud and noisy environment, because mindful eating calls for 100 percent attention to your plate. And, if you have decided to chew your food thoroughly, you need to restrict all other activities and focus only on the meal. The sacrifices are worth it because optimal digestion goes a long way in building a wholesome person.

When I first moved to this country, I was and continue to be intrigued by the regular brown bag meetings at work. In my opinion, these "working lunches" are not the best practice for eating your main meal. You will be forced into participating in several other activities simultaneously: talking, eating, debating, perhaps arguing, and planning. The noise can become an issue, too (e.g., packing and unpacking food, biting on fruits, blowing your nose, etc.). All of this can have a profoundly negative influence on the digestion and absorption of your food. If at all possible, stay away from such meetings, and if you absolutely must attend, refrain from eating during the meeting. Instead, eat before or after the "working lunch."

KITCHEN

My grandfather always claimed, "Optimal health and wellness begins in the kitchen." In fact, the kitchen was considered a sacred place. His home featured a large kitchen with an altar in one small area of the room (see Figure 3 of a modern kitchen with an altar). Throughout the day, I could always count on seeing a member in the kitchen praying, reciting a mantra, lighting a lamp or incense stick, or sounding a bell.

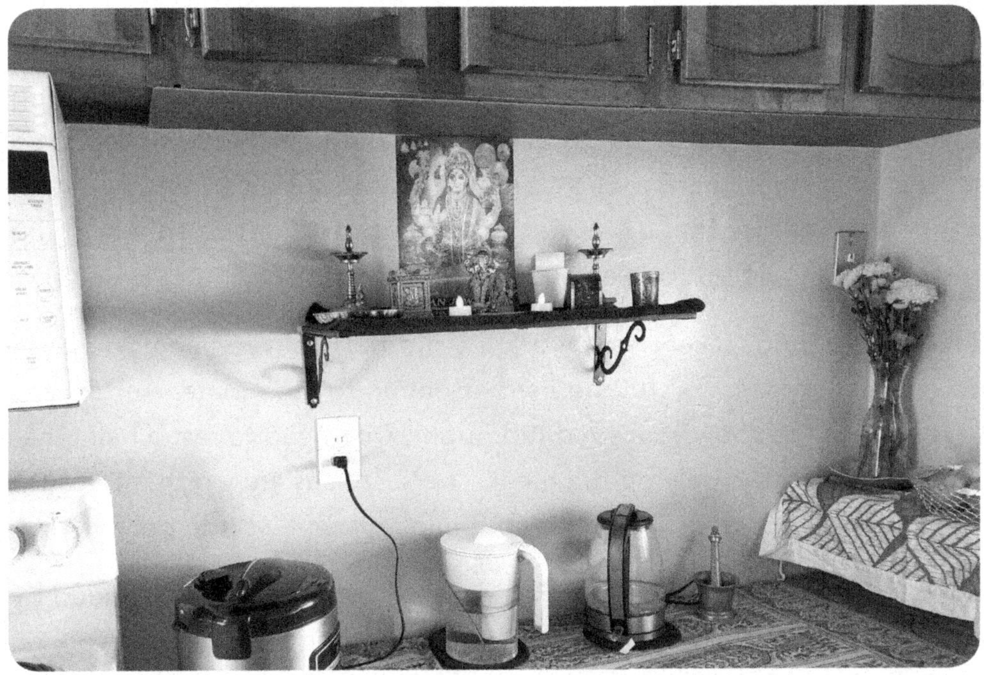

Figure 3: Optimal health and wellness begin in the kitchen. Placing an altar in one corner of the room with a lamp and/or incense and regularly performing devotional recitations there benefits the emotional, mental, and physical status of the family member preparing or eating the food.

The sound vibrations of the mantras, the orange glow from the lamp, and the aromatic smell of the incense kept the emotional and mental prana of the family member preparing the food in high spirits. Then, when we sat down on the floor to eat, the collective mood was positive and calm. The freshly prepared, warm food was rich in prana, and we silently ate.

Another way to raise the prana state is to bring nature into your kitchen by allowing sunlight to stream in the windows, thereby facilitating a bright, safe atmosphere. Decorating your kitchen with potted plants serves as another natural and sustainable home décor that lifts morale and purifies the air (see Figure 4). If you're planning a garden, position it within view of a kitchen window. Watching these plants while preparing or consuming the food is refreshing, calming, and invigorating.

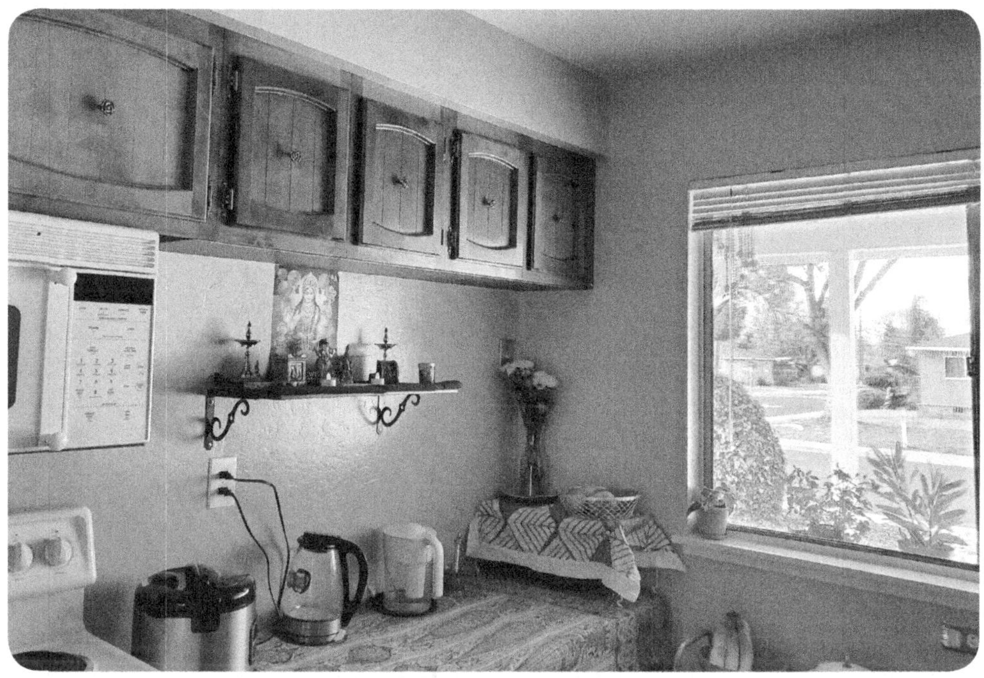

Figure 4: Optimal health and wellness begin in the kitchen. Consider decorating the room with potted plants or allowing sunlight to stream through the windows. This facilitates a bright, safe atmosphere that serves as natural, sustainable home décor, which purifies the air and lifts your morale.

The kitchen should also be free from dirt, trash, and clutter so that it is pleasing to the eye. Ensure that the kitchen walls are painted a warm, attractive color, too. Then, when you enter the kitchen, you will feel relaxed as the sights and smells stimulate your appetite.

A modern-day kitchen is a place of social activity, with people experiencing a wide range of emotions (including those that are not always positive), congregating in the kitchen. Not only that, but people tend to walk straight into the kitchen, wearing their shoes, boots, or sneakers. Giving the bacteria found on our footwear, free access to our kitchen is a cause for concern. Studies show this type of bacteria can trigger intestinal and urinary tract infections, meningitis, and diarrheal disease.[16]

Another hallmark of the modern kitchen is the sheer magnitude of culinary paraphernalia. Despite these tools and gadgets, many people rarely cook in this room. Instead, they heat processed, ready-to-eat food in the microwave and forget silent experiences; eating is almost always accompanied by discussions, phone conversations, or email.

Considering the issues that come with modern kitchen life, it is important to begin holding this space as a revered, sacred room. Do what you can today to transform your kitchen into a place that allows you to explore your true nature and treat yourself as a worthy individual.

CASE STUDY

Gianni entered the restaurant and sat at a small booth toward the front door. After placing his order, he looked around and noticed the rush of cold air every time the front door opened. The noise level in the restaurant was upbeat but loud, and Gianni could barely hear his server describe the daily specials.

The waiter appeared annoyed at the noise as well, rolling his eyes and making comments about how obnoxious people are today. "I can't stand it," the server confided. "People spend so much time on their phones while they eat, but they can't do it quietly! No, they shout into their devices and make it a miserable experience for everyone. I can't wait to get out of this place. Luckily, my shift ends soon."

EATING OUT

A restaurant is another space that we need to consider when eating mindfully. So many of us love to eat in restaurants, but these can be noisy places with many people (and their positive and negative emotions). Restaurant food is often prepared in bulk, and to increase profits, restaurant owners may choose to use cheap, low-prana foods.

If the owner does not treat the staff well and if the hotel staff is disgruntled, they will be preparing your food with negative emotions. All of this results in you paying for the experience of eating low-prana food while consuming other guests' negative emotions. Now, when I visit a restaurant, I always ask the front desk if the chef and the serving staff are in a good mood, and I hesitate to eat there if I suspect the food will be laced with negative emotions. I encourage you, too, to be mindful of where you eat. (Note: If you are traveling, bringing your own food when possible or visiting a local grocery are other viable options to improve your culinary experience.)

You Are WHY You Eat

When asked why we eat, I generally receive one of two responses: "I live to eat," or "I eat to live." The desire to live a long, full life motivates people to seek out and enjoy life's pleasures and pursuits. Scientists have managed to extend life expectancies, and we are constantly pushing aging limits even further. And while longevity may motivate us to eat, there is a higher purpose for sustenance through food.

Albert Einstein once said, "A human being is a spatially and temporally limited piece of the whole, what we call the 'Universe.' He experiences himself and his feelings as separate from the rest, an optical illusion of his consciousness." We need to understand our true nature and who we are at the highest level. Then, we need to use this knowledge and take action that makes the world a better place to live.

A meaningful life is one in which each of us creates something of value that benefits society. To produce something that is of value requires the motivation to pursue and accomplish a worthy goal. Those who are truly conscious of their responsibility to society will never throw away their lives. If souls like Mahatma Gandhi, Mother Teresa, Nelson Mandela, and Martin L. King Jr. can stir the entire world without the backing of politics or money, so can each one of us. But this takes effort and energy, and that cannot be achieved without positive habits, including mindful eating. Thus, when your primary reason for eating is to use food's energy to actively pursue a worthy goal that benefits society, you will find great meaning in your existence and reason for living.

Tips from the GLP Toolbox on Eating Mindfully

Before you eat:

- *Sit in a "high prana" area—a place that is calm, positive, bright, clean, etc.*

- *Silently express gratitude for your meal by thanking nature (for providing an environment that allows crops to grow); farmers (for producing crops); other food workers (responsible for bringing the food from farm to store, restaurant, table, etc.); and the person who prepared the food.*

- *Ensure that you are eating high-prana food. Remember that foods far from their original state in nature only invite health issues and other negative consequences.*

- *If you feel stressed out physically, mentally, or emotionally, first calm your body and mind to prepare for a stress-free dining experience.*

- *For those of you who plan to fast once a month, select the same day each month. For example, if you work, you may wish to choose the first Saturday of each month, while those who stay at home may wish to fast each month on the day of a full moon.*

- *Before you eat your meal, feed three needy people with freshly prepared food (preferably vegetarian) one day each month. This will strengthen the body-mind-emotions nexus*

While you eat:

- *Chew each bite thirty times before swallowing; this count requires you to pay undivided attention to your eating, allowing you to eat mindfully, with a focus.*

- *As you eat, pay attention to your senses to heighten your mindfulness. Notice the colors of the food as well as the textures while chewing. Pay attention to the tastes and smell of each ingredient. Listen to the sound of the food as you chew as well.*

After you eat:

- *Resist eating after your last meal of the day. Do your best to give yourself 12-15 hours between dinner and breakfast.*

Reminder: For optimal results, continue to integrate the practices from this and future chapters into your daily routine. The more practices you can include in your life, the more optimal results you will see!

CHAPTER 2

THE AEROBIC BODY

"From physical exercise, one gets lightness in body and mind, a capacity to work and be stable, enhanced ability to tolerate difficulties, impurities are removed, and the digestive process functions optimally."

CHARAKA SUTRASTHANA–VOL 1.–CHAPTER 7, V32

What do you think of when you hear the word exercise? Many people experience negative associations with the concept of exercise, believing it to be an unenjoyable activity, primarily for young people, and something "extra" you must do for weight management. Some people even believe that older people can't exercise, for fear the activity will exacerbate bone loss and increase the risk of fractures. Unfortunately, only about ten percent of the population above the age of sixty-five engages in a regular physical exercise regimen.[17]

Despite these misconceptions, exercise actually goes a long way to strengthen and protect all parts of the body and brain. In general, aerobics, weight-bearing endurance exercise, resistance exercise, exercises for stability, and exercises that improve balance strengthen the bones, muscles, joints, and vertebrae.[18] Physical exercise stimulates the bone cells and restructures the bone fibers, resulting in more bone mass and improved bone stability,[19] a benefit for young and old alike.

What Happens When We Don't Exercise

While several research studies highlight the benefits of physical exercise, they also discuss the dangers associated with a lack of exercise, sedentary activities, and prolonged sitting. Prolonged sitting and/or sedentary activities are linked to numerous problems, including obesity, high blood pressure, osteoporosis, cardiovascular disease, and colorectal cancer, among others. Prolonged sitting delays fat digestion and metabolism, reduces bone mineral density, and raises the risk of fracture.[20]

Recent research also indicates that prolonged sitting can affect the memory centers in the brain.[21] Simply put, the human body is not built to sit for long periods. Our ancestors—the hominin—naturally spent many hours outdoors, walking, hunting, and foraging for food. Physical exercise to these cavemen was not considered "working out," but instead just a part of daily living. Compare this to our modern world, where physical activity is considered an intervention, something we do to prevent the negative consequences that result from a sedentary lifestyle.

But what if you exercise daily, before or after a long day at your sedentary job? Scientists warn that prolonged sitting for eight hours or longer offsets any benefits that come from daily exercise.[22] This suggests that, even if you fulfill the recommended guidelines for daily exercise, you are still at a higher risk for disease and declining health.

Is the solution to spend more time standing? While it is true that too much standing can affect the legs, knees, and lower back, most experts recommend a fifty-fifty sit-stand balance for optimal health.[23]

So, what could this look like in the real world? Because I spend many hours sitting at a desk, I like to interrupt my sitting time as often as possible. I try to do this by moving or stretching for at least ten minutes for every hour that I sit at the desk.

What Happens When We Exercise

Now, let's turn to what happens when we *do* exercise by taking an in-depth look at its benefits.

WEIGHT LOSS

Physical exercise can help control weight. Excess weight or obesity results from an energy imbalance and intake of excess calories with too few calories being burnt. While several factors determine energy expenditure, like age, body size, or genes, the most easily modified factor is physical activity. Having a regular regimen of physical exercise helps a person to maintain a healthy weight. Researchers are still uncertain about just how much activity people need each day to maintain a healthy weight or to help with weight loss. However, researchers unanimously believe that regular physical exercise is a useful lifestyle practice for weight management. The more active people are, the more likely they are to maintain their weight.

The Women's Health Study, which followed more than 30,000 middle-aged women for thirteen years, found that women needed the equivalent of one hour a day of moderate-to-vigorous physical activity to maintain a steady weight.[24] The *type* of activity also made a difference: bicycling and brisk walking helped women avoid weight gain. Similarly, in another trial involving 320 post-menopausal women, researchers noticed that forty-five minutes of moderate-to-vigorous aerobic activity, five days a week, resulted in the exercise group experiencing significant decreases in body weight, body fat, and abdominal fat, compared to the control (non-exercising) group.[25]

Physical activity boosts total energy expenditure, decreases fat around the waist and total body fat, and reduces depression and anxiety, which motivates us to continue our exercise regimens over time.[26]

HEART HEALTH

Our overall health is dependent upon the heart's ability to pump blood to all of our organs, regardless of the body's fluctuating external and internal environment.

As with other muscles, the heart muscles become strong when they contract and relax repeatedly through exercise. Not only that, but just as flossing removes plaque and food particles under the gums and between the teeth, physical exercise flosses out (or burns away) fat deposits that accumulate in the blood vessels. This allows the blood to flow smoothly and draw in more oxygen.

Studies have also shown that exercise helps the blood vessels to sprout and branch out, creating new bypass routes for the blood to travel if the normal path is blocked by fat deposits. In addition, exercise increases the levels of good cholesterol (HDL) in the body. All of this adds up to a decreased risk of heart disease thanks to a stronger heart, better blood circulation, increased oxygen levels, lower blood pressure, and improved lipid profiles.[27]

MANAGEMENT OF DIABETES

In addition to reducing the risk of heart disease, regular physical exercise optimizes blood sugar and insulin levels, thereby reducing one's risk of diabetes.[28]

FORTIFIES BONES AND MUSCLES

Regular exercise strengthens bones and muscles and delays age-associated bone density loss. Muscle-strengthening exercises increase and/or sustain muscle mass and strength, too.[29]

IMPROVES SLEEP

Exercise improves sleep quality. People who incorporate exercise into their daily lifestyle agree that it helps them to fall asleep faster and stay asleep longer.[30]

INCREASES LONGEVITY

Studies show that physical activity can increase your health span (years spent with no illness).[31]

REDUCES INFLAMMATION

Inflammation is an important physiological response of the body's immune system. It is the body's effort to defend itself against toxic invaders like viruses and bacteria. It is also the body's response to repair damaged tissue or heal after an injury.

On occasions, these defense molecules turn haywire, thinking its own tissue is foreign. When this happens, the body begins attacking itself, which leads to chronic inflammation, an underlying feature of several serious health issues, including diabetes, celiac disease, obesity, arthritis, thyroid disease, neuritis, tendonitis, and other conditions. Fortunately, several scientific studies have demonstrated that moderate exercise can suppress and even reverse chronic inflammation.[32]

IMPROVES BRAIN HEALTH

I believe in the adage that "what is good for the heart is good for the brain as well, and vice versa." In addition to its beneficial effects on the heart and body in general, physical exercise also has a positive impact on mental and emotional health in the following ways:

- **REVERSES NEGATIVE MOODS**

  Physical exercise stimulates the release of several feel-good neurochemicals that mitigate mood disorders, including fear, worry, anxiety, and depression. Studies also demonstrate that exercise helps us overcome depressive symptoms associated with major depressive disorder.[33]

- **INCREASES CEREBRAL BLOOD FLOW**

  Physical exercise increases blood flow, resulting in more oxygen to the brain. Increased cerebral blood flow brings with it vital nutrients and more fuel for the brain to function optimally.[34]

- **PROTECTS AND STIMULATES NEW BRAIN CELLS**

  Physical exercise activates several brain-specific genes with neuroprotective properties. These neurochemicals protect the brain cells from toxins and other deterrents, as well as supporting the production of brain cells that provide the structural framework and wiring for the brain.[35]

One such neurochemical is called BDNF (brain-derived neurotrophic factor). This neurochemical supports the survival of existing neurons, strengthens nerve-to-nerve communication, and, in some cases, stimulates the growth and differentiation of new neuronal cells.[35]

- **DELAYS THE ONSET OF DEMENTIA**

  Several studies show that regular aerobic activity leads to structural changes in the brain that delay or even reverse memory loss. While the risk for dementia and Alzheimer's disease depends on several factors, including genetics, dietary choices, stress, sleep quality, and activity levels, it is still incredibly important to exercise to maintain optimal brain function.[36]

  Some studies report that for those with mild to moderate cognitive impairment, thirty minutes of daily exercise that includes endurance activities, strength training, balance, and flexibility will not only improve their physical health but also cognitive function. Moderate-to-high levels of physical exercise have beneficial effects on the brain as well, especially as it relates to executive function (which assists with self-regulation, planning, focus, etc.) in middle-aged and older adults.[37]

- **REGULATES THE HPA AXIS**

  The HPA (hypothalamic–pituitary–adrenal) axis involves the hypothalamus (the master gland), the pituitary (a pea-sized structure located below the hypothalamus), and the adrenal glands (small organs on top of the kidneys). This triumvirate acts in sync to regulate mood, emotions, cognition, digestion, metabolism, energy, and the immune system. Physical exercise stabilizes and resets the HPA axis, thereby improving physical, mental, and emotional health.[38]

Getting Started

You now understand the benefits of exercise, but you still may not know how to get started. This section will help. First, physical exercise is not something that you must do only at a gym or fitness facility. You don't need to spend a lot of money to be fit. In fact, you can get in shape from the comfort of your home! Best of all, when you adopt a fitness mindset, you'll begin finding ways to incorporate physical activity throughout your entire day. This is good news because studies suggest that a reasonable amount of activity, particularly during the middle and later years, effectively lowers the risk of serious illness, improves the quality of life, and adds more years to your life.[39]

Choose whatever type of exercise suits you best and engage in that regimen daily. Consider solo activities like walking and running, team sports and leagues (think tennis, golf, soccer, etc.), and outdoor activities such as hiking, skiing, and swimming. If you enjoy group classes and you decide you do want to join a gym, you may choose to sign up for anything from yoga and Pilates to Zumba and spinning. Take time to determine which physical activities attract and keep you comfortable. Remember, it should not stress you out. Rather, exercise that is the right fit for you should leave you in a high-prana state, pleasant, and even perhaps euphoric.

Here are some additional exercise suggestions:

ENDURANCE EXERCISES

Endurance exercises make you breathe harder and increase your heart rate. This includes brisk walking, dancing, cycling, running, and swimming.

RESISTANCE OR STRENGTH-TRAINING EXERCISES

These exercises work all the major muscle groups of the body and improve bone strength, muscle strength, and muscular fitness. Activities include weight lifting, push-ups, pull-ups, crunches, and squats.

YOGA

Yoga asanas (poses) increase muscle strength, power, and endurance through specific strength training poses. By holding the body in specific poses, you will improve your balance, strength, flexibility, agility, and stamina. Sun salutations, inversions, and forward bending poses (with yoga breath practices) optimize your blood pressure and heart rate as well.

Breath practice is an integral part of yoga, performed in sync with inhalation and exhalation. This increases lung capacity and promotes the delivery of oxygen to the body. The increased flow of oxygen helps with overall performance and efficiency, relieves soreness, and enhances tissue repair.

There are a variety of yoga poses that will loosen tight hips, improve the range of motion and circulation, and resolve any leg or low back pain. For these poses, the emphasis is on the back, lateral side, and front hip.

INVERSIONS

Inversions require the heart to be positioned above the head—a natural way to stimulate blood flow to the brain, increase circulation throughout the entire body, and counter the effects of gravity on the skeletal system.

If you are a beginner, there are props, such as inversion tables, that will help you achieve the proper position. Furthermore, if you are in a class setting, it is always advantageous to receive proper guidance from a trained teacher who can suggest the correct way to move into and sustain the inversion pose. The teacher's guidance will help a student move into the pose and find his or her balance. With manual adjustments from the teacher, you may achieve better stability, as well as the ability to go deeper into the pose.

FLEXIBILITY EXERCISES

Flexibility exercises include anything involving stretching and bending, and they will improve your range of motion and overall mobility. For example, a Pilates workout builds strength, but it also boosts your flexibility and joint mobility.

HIP ABDUCTION EXERCISES

The hips (pelvis) are a collection of the two hip bones (ilia), the last part of the spinal cord (sacrum), and other ligaments and muscles, which provide stability, strength, and motion to the pelvis. As we age, our hips become weak and susceptible to damage, either due to excessive motion or lack of motion. The tighter our hips, the less flexible our lower back and upper spine become, making it difficult to walk, sit, or stand. That's why hip abduction exercises are great for men and women of all ages.[40]

How Much Exercise is Enough?

You may now be asking how much physical activity is required to achieve remarkable change. Studies indicate that at least twenty minutes daily (of moderate exercise) or ten minutes a day (of vigorous exercise) is the minimum requirement to reap the overall benefits.[41] Please note that if your motive is to lose weight or fulfill more rigorous fitness goals, you will most likely need to do even more than twenty minutes daily.

CASE STUDY

Mary, a resident of the San Francisco Bay area, works as a consultant for a reputable financial firm in New York City. Her work required her to travel each week to New York City. This resulted in weekly travels, changes in routines, irregular meals, disruption of her body's circadian rhythms, and poor sleep. Mary's schedule also prevented her from engaging in any physical activity. Within a few years of this routine, Mary's health suffered. At first, Mary refused to follow any of my suggestions since she did not "have time" to implement any recommendations.

However, when her health issues became more serious, she approached me again with one request: she would follow just one lifestyle change. Knowing that she lived close to a park, I asked her to take a walk barefoot in the park for at least one hour daily or whenever her schedule permitted.

Mary incorporated this change and went for her walks regularly (except for the days when she was on the East Coast). Soon, she noticed that some of her health issues improved, and she felt more energetic. That one change encouraged her to adopt additional changes, including eating freshly-cooked meals at home. A combination of the "grounded physical activity" coupled with a fresh high prana diet added even more cheer and vitality to her life.

To benefit fully from exercise, get into the habit of engaging in vigorous and moderate endurance exercises along with strength and flexibility exercises. You do not need to accomplish this in a single workout. For example, you could begin your day with stretching, followed by an endurance activity. Later on, you could engage in some strength exercises. Or, you might choose to alternate activities throughout the week.

For someone who simply does not like to exercise, I would suggest engaging in some light physical activity that is enjoyable, offers variety, and is appropriate for his or her age. If you are still unsure or confused about where or how to start, follow some of the tips provided at the end of this section as a substitute for a daily physical exercise. Consider the case of Mary to learn how you, too, can fit exercise into a busy lifestyle even if you don't currently exercise.

A Gentle Reminder

Please remember, along with exercise, it is still important to eat mindfully to see true benefits. Interestingly, research studies have shown that exercise and fasting both trigger the production and activation of several "feel good" chemicals in the body that strengthen and nourish the body, mind, and emotions. Activating these chemicals through exercise and fasting can help ward off illness, as well as minimize the consequences of chronic health conditions.[42]

Personally, I have found a routine that works best for me: fasting overnight for at least twelve hours, followed by forty-five minutes of moderate exercise the next morning, and then followed by a light breakfast. This kick-starts the production of the feel-good chemicals in a natural way, and I have found that this helps me maintain a balanced state of body, mind, and emotions.

Tips from the GLP Toolbox for the Aerobic Body

If you don't feel you have the time for daily exercise, try some of these ideas to begin incorporating activity into your normal routine:

- *If you spend any time outdoors, incorporate grounding into your day. Grounding refers to direct body contact with the earth's surface (soil, sand, or water). Several evidence-based research studies indicate that grounding reverses pain and inflammation.*[43] *Some simple ways to ground yourself include hiking in nature, walking barefoot on the beach or in the grass, gardening, or engaging in other yard work without using gloves.*

- *During a break at work or while watching television, bend your knees and sit or squat on the floor. Remain in this position for fifteen seconds, and then rise to a standing position, using as little support as possible. If you complete this sequence at least nine times, it only takes five minutes or so to increase your mobility, flexibility, and functional capabilities.*

- *While watching television, engage in some light stretching, twisting, and lifting.*

- *Instead of using a vacuum cleaner, use a broom. This works your hips, spine, wrists, and even your elbows and knees since cleaning under tables and chairs may require you to squat and bend low to the ground.*

- *If you sit for long periods at work, consider investing in a standing desk. Then, for every thirty minutes you sit, stand and work for thirty minutes. You can set an alarm on your phone or computer to remind you when it's time to stand or sit.*

- *If possible, walk or bike to work. If the distance is too far, determine if it's possible to drive part of the way, and then walk or bike the remainder of the distance.*

- *Whenever possible, take the stairs instead of the elevator.*

- *During long meetings, make a point to stand midway through the meeting. Better yet, attempt to arrange walking meetings!*

- *Park your car as far from the door of your work or a store as possible.*

- *Instead of emailing someone at work, walk to that person to ask your question.*

Reminder: For optimal results, continue to integrate the practices from all previous and future chapters into your daily routine. The more practices you can include in your life, the more optimal results you will see!

CHAPTER 3

TUNING THE BODY

"May my life breathe, all my limbs, sense faculties (sound, touch, sight, taste and smell) be abound and prosper so I realize my true nature."

PEACE MANTRA – KENA UPANISHAD

You take your vehicle to the mechanic for maintenance to avoid problems down the road. The mechanic then employs a standard operating procedure (SOP) to check, clean, and/or replace the various parts if needed. That's because a car that does not undergo regular maintenance is more prone to mechanical problems. Driving a poorly maintained car invites serious trouble since you cannot predict when the brakes, engine, or other components will break down. To prevent emergencies like this, your mechanic might suggest periodic tune-ups to identify potential problems before they turn into bigger issues. This is to play it safe and avoid situations that can put your life in danger.

Now, let's apply this concept to your body. When was the last time that you gave your body a tune-up? Our bodies are more specialized and complex than a car, yet there are some similarities when it comes to tuning and maintenance. For instance, regular self-care and tuning of the body are necessary as a preventative measure to head off serious health issues and to live an optimal life. So just as the auto mechanic uses an SOP to check oil, filters, drive belts, fluids, tire pressure, and treads, we need an SOP that will help us tune-up and maintain the five sense organs to benefit the body, brain, and emotions.

The five sense organs are the ears, skin, eyes, tongue, and nose. You use your five senses to draw in external information, and then translate what you objectively experience into a subjective response. In other words, if you take in healthy, positive impressions through your senses, your subjective response will be to experience feelings of happiness and harmony.

According to Ayurveda and Yoga texts, the intake of harmonious sensory impressions through the five senses results in a positive state of health and well being. However, if we absorb unhealthy impressions through the five senses, we may suffer and fall prey to health issues and premature medical problems. A simple way to avoid misery and discomfort, then, is to continually "tune" your five sense organs:

Ears

The ear receives sound waves from the outside world, and those sound waves are amplified in the middle ear. These waves are then converted into nerve impulses, which are transferred to specific areas of the brain. The brain converts these impulses into a perceivable sound wave.

This progression of sound is important because what we hear will affect our emotions, mind, and physical body. If the sounds are pleasant, those feel-good chemicals will be released in our bodies, and we will experience positive feelings.

Some common sounds that are part of our daily lives include noise from the road, rail, and air traffic; occupational and industrial noise; sounds from nature; and music, television, and video sounds. All of these sounds impact the ears and health, for better or for worse.

Words are also sounds, and they have their own subtle energies that can profoundly affect the recipient. While curse words will negatively affect the person hearing them, loving words of encouragement will have an uplifting, positive effect. The key to good health and wellness, then, is to do our best to expose our ears to pleasant, motivating sounds.

Your ears also play a major role in the sense of balance and body position, thanks to the mastoids, which are bony projections behind the ear. They are responsible for moment-to-moment monitoring of the position and movement of the head to create stability and balance.

TUNING AND MAINTENANCE

Follow the suggestions below to tune and protect the ears (and sense of hearing):

- **YOGA**

  Karna Mastiska Yoga, based on the principle of ear acupuncture and the body's subtle energy system, is a simple and effective technique to energize and recharge the brain. Pilot studies on the effects of Karna Mastiska Yoga (also referred to as Super Brain Yoga) showed significant increases in academic and behavioral performance, greater class participation, improved social skills, and increased electrical activity in the brain.[44]

  The Karna Mastiska Yoga technique involves crossing the arms, holding the earlobes, and squatting. First, take your left hand and hold your right earlobe with your thumb and forefinger, with the thumb in front. Then, take your right hand and cross it over your left elbow to hold your left earlobe in the same way. At this point, you should be applying pressure to both earlobes simultaneously.

  As you hold this pose, inhale through your nose, and bend your knees as you gently squat down to the ground. Hold the pose for two-to-five seconds, and then exhale as you start making your way back to a standing position. Repeat this technique nine times.

  Interestingly, in my native country of India, one of the punishments meted out to misbehaving kids at home or at school was Karna Mastiska Yoga. The child would move to a time-out corner of the room and perform a few rounds of this exercise. In hindsight, I wonder if the punishment's purpose was to improve the sense of hearing so the child could better focus on books and studies.

- **OLEATION**

  This preventative technique involves intra-auricular application ("Karna Purana" in Ayurveda) of warm coconut, sesame, almond, or olive oil. In addition to maintaining ear health, oleation treats ear infections, dryness or itching in the ears, tinnitus (ear ringing), neck/jaw tension, headaches, and wax or yeast overgrowth. (This is according to Ayurveda and these health claims are not supported by evidence from scientific studies).

It is convenient to use a fluid dropper to apply one to two drops of oil into each ear. Tilt the neck to one side and dispense two drops of the oil into the ear. Wait ten seconds, and then repeat this sequence in the other ear by tilting the neck on the opposite side. After completing this procedure, close your eyes and gently bring your neck forward. Relax before proceeding with the next therapy.

- **LISTENING TO THE SOUNDS OF NATURE**

  Sit in a comfortable position in the garden, park, or by a water pond. Close your eyes and pay attention to the sounds of nature. Let go of all other dramas in your mind and just concentrate on the sounds around you as you inhale and exhale. If you find that your mind is wandering, simply release those thoughts and bring your focus back to the sounds of nature. Do this for thirty minutes daily (or on the weekends at a minimum).

- **LISTENING TO YOUR INNER VOICE**

  In addition to physical sounds, your sense of sound also involves paying attention to your inner voice. This is the voice of the mind and emotions that many consider a trustworthy source of accuracy and truth. When you choose to listen to your inner voice and allow it to guide you, you will quickly recognize your own unconscious biases and assumptions. As you become more attuned to your inner voice, you will develop a sense of inner knowing that is wise and true. Spend time each day noticing and becoming more aware of this inner voice that helps guide your thoughts, actions, and decisions.

A WORD OF CAUTION

Between headphones and Bluetooth-enabled earbuds, wireless devices that cover the ears have become extremely common. Unfortunately, the radiation emitted from these devices is an unintended yet serious side effect. Several patients who see me for Ayurveda treatments complain of frequent headaches and/or unusual ear pain. I have found that these are usually the same people who frequently use wireless communication devices in their ears.

Although the FDA declares that research studies have failed to show an association between exposure to these devices and health issues, I always recommend moderate use. And if you're willing to restrict your use altogether, even better!

If you tune your ears regularly and avoid the wireless ear devices you're sure to notice improvements to your sense of hearing, while developing a greater appreciation of how your ears serve you.

Skin

As the largest external organ, the skin has many functions, but the primary one is to perceive the sense of touch. Thanks to the skin, we can experience variations in temperature, pressure, and pain. The skin is densely packed with nerve cells and constantly communicates with the brain. This sensory stimulation is what causes you to offer a handshake, reach out for a hug, or even fight back by slapping or beating.

Have you ever noticed how a simple massage leaves you smiling and feeling relaxed? Or how a bear hug calms you down? While meaningful touches evoke pleasant feelings, other sensations your skin perceives can feel unpleasant and stressful. In other words, your response is dependent on what your skin perceives from the outside world.

The skin also insulates the entire body, guarding it against extreme temperature, harsh sunlight, toxic pollutants, and chemicals. It protects the body from persistent infection and is a site of synthesis of vitamin D (an important vitamin that helps maintain healthy bones and teeth; supports the health of the immune, brain, lung, and cardiovascular systems; and protects against chronic inflammatory conditions).[45]

Unfortunately, due to modern yet unhealthy living conditions and lifestyle practices, recent reports suggest that a significant percentage of the world population is at an increased risk of skin cancer or premature skin aging (including unhealthy skin) due to suboptimal levels of vitamin D.[46]

For your mind and emotions, the sense of touch allows you to feel a connection to everything around you and become aware of your feelings, intentions, and disposition. This sense also extends to touching the lives of others and making a difference in the world. Therefore, our touch needs to be an inspiration to those around us, so that our lives—and the lives of others—become meaningful and worthwhile.

TUNING AND MAINTENANCE

The tips below will allow you to tune and maintain your skin, and they can be done daily, weekly, or monthly:

- **BATH PRODUCTS**

  Try to avoid using soaps or shampoos made from synthetic chemicals. Instead, create a thin, water-based paste of lavender, jasmine, or rose bath salts. Scrub this lightly over your wet skin in the shower, and then rinse off and pat dry.

- **MASSAGE OIL**

  Make massage oil by mixing one-half ounce of coconut oil and one-half ounce of almond oil together in a bottle. Add ten drops of lavender, jasmine, or rose essential oil to the mixture, and then warm the bottle in hot water for a few minutes.

Pour some oil onto your palms and massage your scalp, the tops and bottoms of the feet, abdomen, back, and the rest of your body. Use circular strokes on the joints, and long and repetitive strokes on your limbs and bony areas. This home practice allows you to appreciate and love your skin and other tissues. Also, note how this procedure calms the mind and senses.

Eyes

The eyes are the most beautiful and expressive organs. Together with the brain, the eyes are responsible for converting visual impulses to electrical signals via the optic nerve. These signals are then processed in specific areas of the brain, resulting in our ability to see and appreciate shapes, sizes, colors, and objects in a three-dimensional world.[47]

Our eyes are also responsible for our perception of self, constantly reminding us of our true nature and close connection with the universe. Through our sense of sight, we "see" and appreciate the divine that is present within us and in our outside world. This results in our ability to know our true nature, purpose in life, and the contributions we can make to society and humanity.

TUNING AND MAINTENANCE

To fully appreciate the eyes and the perception of sight, we need to do everything we can to keep our eyes and vision perfect and healthy:

- **EYE EXERCISES**

  Exercising the eyes daily is a simple way to strengthen them and ward off ocular disease. One simple method is to move your eyeballs right and left, upwards and downwards, and then rotate them in clockwise and counterclockwise directions.

- **PALMING**

  For this method of bringing relief to the eyes, rub your palms vigorously to generate heat, and then slightly cup your palms and place them over the eyes. When the warmth subsides, remove your palms and repeat the procedure. According to Ayurveda, this exercise helps achieve proper vision, sharpens the ability to discriminate colors, and enhances perception.

- **INTRAOCULAR MASSAGE (*NETRA BASTI*)**

  Otherwise known as IOM, netra basti is a restorative and preventative Ayurveda technique for the eyes. There are two simple ways to perform it:

  Option 1: Dip your index finger into ghee, coconut oil, or sesame oil and apply it to the inside corner of one eyelid. Move the oil across the eyelid to the outer corner. Repeat with the other index finger to the second eye and repeat the stroke pattern.

  Option 2: Fill a glass eye cup with warm oil. Lean over and press the cup over the eye, making sure the cup creates a tight fit. Slowly straighten your head and tilt it back as you continue pressing the cup against your eye. Gently open your eye and look through the oil for sixty seconds. Lower your head and neck and carefully remove the cup. Repeat this process with your other eye.

  An intraocular massage can help reduce stress, tension, or migraine headaches; delay age-associated degeneration of the eyes; improve vision; and strengthen the nervous system. These benefits based on Ayurveda texts are not supported by evidence from scientific studies.

- **LAMP GAZING (*TRATAKA*)**

  This is the practice of staring at the orange glow of a burning candle or oil wick without blinking. As you fix your gaze on the glow, pay attention to each thought and feeling. Notice those thoughts and feelings, and then gently let them go. Allow yourself to become completely absorbed in the flame's glow, and continue staring until your eyes begin to water. At this point, close your eyes and relax. This exercise will help to strengthen your eyes, as well as improve your focus and concentration.

SOME WORDS OF CAUTION

To better protect your eye health:

- *Avoid staying up late at night and sleeping past sunrise, as this is harmful to the eyes.*[48] *Instead, adjust your routine to retire earlier and awake with the sun. And when you wake up each day, splash cool water into your eyes around five times.*

- *Be sure to follow the dietary guidelines in Chapter 1 to ensure that you have regular bowel movements, as constipation can actually weaken eyesight.*[49]

- *Avoid emotional turbulence, including worry, anxiety, grief, and anger. These emotions can be harmful to the eyes.*[50]

- *Cultivate a habit of blinking or resting the eyes. Staring continuously, especially while viewing objects at a distance, is not good for your eye health.*[51]

- *Avoid staring at objects in bright sunlight for a long period of time.*

- *Avoid reading, writing, or working with your eyes in poor light or when the light is not sufficient.*

- *Try to shield your eyes from dust and smoke, since these are harmful pollutants to the eye.*[51]

Nose

The nose is the gateway to the sense of smell. Flavors, aromas, fragrances, and even unpleasant smells are just some of the olfactory stimuli detected by the nose. When you recognize a specific smell, these odorants (smell-stimulating substances) bind to olfactory receptors in your nasal cavity. The signals from these receptors are then transmitted to the olfactory lobes in your brain, which then processes these signals to generate a suitable response. And as one of the oldest and most vital parts of the brain, the olfactory lobes also influence your emotions, behavior, and memory.

Because smells are closely associated with emotions, certain smells will evoke long-forgotten memories of special occasions, both positive and negative. I clearly remember an episode of this during an Ayurveda nutrition class. During the class, I asked each student to open a small Ziploc bag that contained a spice. One of the bags contained the spice asafoetida, which has a noxious, sulfurous smell. When one of the students opened the bag, another student began vomiting. Now, fast-forward three years. I was coaching some Ayurveda students, and this same student sat in my class. As we discussed ways to correct digestive imbalances, I suggested a mix of spices with the chief spice being asafoetida. When I mentioned that spice, the student's brain made the connection to this memory, and she immediately began vomiting again—even without smelling the actual spice!

In addition to the smell-memory connection, the sense of smell is closely associated with the sense of taste.[52] This is evident when a person who suffers from colds loses not only the sense of smell but also the ability to taste food. Therefore, to fully appreciate your sense of smell and its affiliation to memories and taste, you will want to follow the suggestions below to keep your nose as perfect and healthy as possible.

TUNING AND MAINTENANCE

These nasal therapies are natural methods to keep your nasal passages clear and functioning properly:

- **NASAL CLEANSING**

  Known as jala neti in Sanskrit, nasal cleansing is a cost-effective, drug-free, and all-natural technique that is believed to prevent respiratory ailments and clear out any toxins from the nasal passage.

  This is accomplished by using a neti pot, which has been around for centuries, originating with the Ayurveda/Yoga medical tradition. Its popularity and usage are on the rise in the U.S. as well.

  This technique involves filling the specialized neti pot with filtered warm water and combining it with a quarter teaspoon of non-iodized salt. Stir the water with a spoon so that the salt is completely dissolved, and then ensure that the water temperature is tolerable by dipping your finger into the pot.

  Turn your head to the side and insert the neti pot spout into your upper nostril, allowing the salt water to flow into it. Breathe out of your mouth to relax as you do this. If your head posture is correct, the saline solution will begin pouring out of the lower nostril. Keep your chin tucked under, as this will prevent the salt water from going down your throat.

When done correctly, there is no discomfort because the temperature of the water is close to your body temperature, and the salinity of the water is the same as the interior of your nasal passageway. After finishing with one nostril, repeat the procedure on the other side. When you're finished, remove any remaining water from the nose by slowly folding forward and turning your head from side to side.

- **NASYA KARMA**

  Another nasal therapy advocated by the Ayurveda medical tradition that is also of interest in modern medicine is nasya karma. This therapy involves administering herbal oils, herbal powders, or liquid medicines through the nostrils.

  Using a small glass pipet with a rubber bulb, tilt your head and neck back slightly, and dispense two drops of either coconut, sesame, olive, or sunflower oil into one nostril. Close the other nostril with the forefinger and inhale three times to allow the oil to go deep into the nasal cavity. Repeat the same in the other nostril. After completing this procedure, close your eyes and gently bring your neck forward.

  The therapy is believed to cleanse and open the sinuses and channels of the brain to improve oxygenation, which directly influences brain function. Ayurveda recommends this technique to cure headaches, dry nose and voice, nervousness, anxiety, fear, dizziness, conjunctivitis, and any nasal infection.

  It is worth noting that nasya therapy is becoming popular in modern medicine as well because of its ability to help treat neurodegenerative conditions. Typically, oral intake of drugs is by far the most commonly used and desirable route for their delivery since they reach the systemic areas through the bloodstream. However, because this type of delivery does not allow the drugs to reach the brain, treatment for brain conditions is challenging.

The brain is endowed with a blood-brain-barrier (BBB) that prevents the entry of a large number of molecules, including drugs that are being delivered. Breaching the BBB is not a good option, as it would facilitate the entry of toxins and other undesirable molecules into the brain, resulting in more damage.

Attempts were made to override the barrier by other novel and non-invasive approaches, and nasya therapy proved useful because of a lack of an effective barrier between the nasal cavity and the olfactory region of the brain. Compounds introduced into the nasal cavity find their way directly to different regions of the brain, eliminating the need for systemic delivery.[53] *Thus, combining the experiential wisdom of Ayurveda with empirical advances from modern medical science provides non-invasive, faster, better, and more affordable therapies for brain conditions via the nose.*

Tongue

The cells that respond to taste are known as gustatory cells. These cells make up the taste buds, which are located primarily on the upper surface of the tongue. When it comes to your sense of taste, the chemical particles in food bind to taste receptors on the taste buds, which stimulate associated nerves, eventually carrying the information to the brain.

Ayurveda texts describe six major taste sensations including: sweet, salt, sour, bitter, pungent, and astringent. Because these taste (and smell) sensations decrease in sensitivity as we grow older,[54] regular tuning and maintenance of the tongue and mouth are necessary to sustain your taste response.

TUNING AND MAINTENANCE

No matter your age, it's never too early to work on maintaining a healthy tongue to optimize your sense of taste:

- **TONGUE CLEANING**

  According to Ayurveda, optimal digestion—the foundation of good health and wellness—begins in the mouth when food first comes into contact with the tongue. Cleansing the tongue enhances the sense of taste and supports the entire digestive process. A coating on the tongue indicates the presence of toxins, and this contributes to improper digestion. Not only that, but the accumulation of the cellular debris and toxins on the tongue are the main causes of halitosis (bad breath) and other common health problems.

  Scientific studies show that 80-95 percent of bad breath cases originate mainly from material on the rear of the tongue. This stuff also contributes to periodontal problems, plaque on the teeth, tooth decay, gum infections, gum recession, and tooth loss.[55]

  A tongue cleaner (also called a tongue scraper or tongue brush) is an oral hygiene device designed to clear the coating and cellular debris from the surface of the tongue. This gently removes the toxins from the tongue while stimulating and cleansing the associated organs and deep tissues. According to Ayurveda, the tongue serves as a road map of the entire body, with each section of the tongue corresponding to a specific organ. Thus, it is a good practice to clean the surface of the tongue at least once daily with a tongue cleaner. Adding this practice to your daily routine eliminates toxins from the body, massages and strengthens the internal organs, and stimulates digestion.[56]

Ideally, you should clean your tongue early in the morning on an empty stomach, using a stainless steel U- or V-shaped scraper. The use of any other device can be risky, resulting in injuries to the tongue or taste buds.

Hold the ends of the tongue scraper in both hands, stick the tongue out, and place the tongue scraper on the surface of the tongue as far back as it can go. Gently pull the tongue scraper forward so that it removes the coating on the tongue. Repeat the process three times. Each stroke needs to be gentle so as not to harm the underlying tissue, yet vigorous enough to remove the coating. Tip: Relaxing the tongue helps to avoid the gag reflex or vomiting.

- **CHEWING BITTER HERBS**

  Ayurveda recommends bitter-tasting herbs to nourish the taste buds, gums and teeth, due to their antimicrobial properties. Chewing one end of the twig, stem, or root of the bitter plants helps to fight bad breath, prevent infections, improve salivation, reduce hunger, and flush out toxins from the mouth.

  After chewing one end of the twig, stem, or root, use the bristles like a brush to clean your teeth. If you reside in India or the Indian subcontinent, bitter herbs would include neem (Azadirachta indica) or guduchi (Tinospora cordifolia). If you happen to live in the West, you can use chamomile, dandelion, or burdock.

- **OIL PULLING** *(GANDUSHA)*

  As part of the daily routine (and a good practice), this technique involves swishing cold-pressed oil or refined oil in the mouth in the morning on an empty stomach.[57]

Take one teaspoon of oil in the mouth and, without swallowing, move, rinse, swish, suck, and pull the oil slowly through the teeth for two to five minutes. Continue the process until the oil has gotten thinner and loses its original color through mixing with the saliva. If the oil has not changed color, it has not been pulled long enough.

After swishing sufficiently, spit the oil into a trash bin and rinse your mouth with warm water. Swishing activates the salivary enzymes that help to draw out cellular debris and other toxins. Ayurveda recommends this technique to optimize digestion, improve cellular metabolism, and to sustain good health.

I have used coconut, sesame, sunflower, ghee, and olive oil for the past fifteen years, and I have not had any oral issues. In fact, my dentist complains that my teeth are boring since they do not require any additional work or cost for him to correct.

Tips from the GLP Toolbox on Tuning the Body

Keep in mind that regular maintenance of the five senses facilitates good quality sleep, promotes nerve branching, and strengthens the brain-body nexus. By starting gradually with a few of the suggestions from this chapter, you can begin to incorporate some healthy practices into your routine that will contribute to better health, as well as a reduction in symptoms you may currently be experiencing. Take a closer look at the changes a former student noticed in her life after using just a few of these practices:

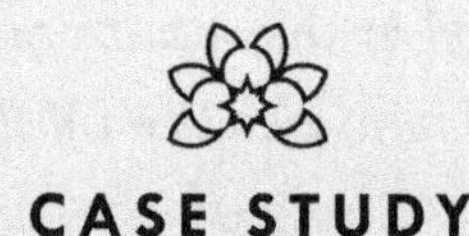

CASE STUDY

When Rashida came to me for relief from her sinus and digestive issues, she was experiencing multiple bothersome symptoms, from indigestion and nighttime coughing to an ongoing postnasal drip. Rashida had become accustomed to a regimen of both prescription and over-the-counter remedies. While the medications provided some relief, she did not like the idea of becoming dependent on them; however, whenever she tried to stop using a medication, the symptoms would almost immediately return.

Rashida started to gradually incorporate some of the practices from this chapter to help. First, she began using the neti pot in the morning and evening to clear her nasal passages, allowing her to breathe freely. Occasionally, she would use nasya therapy in lieu of the neti pot. She then introduced oil pulling into her morning routine, along with tongue scraping.

Within several weeks, Rashida returned to my office. "The postnasal drip has almost completely disappeared, and that's reduced the coughing at night!" she told me excitedly. "Not only that, but I've cut way back on the antacids. I think the tongue scraping and oil pulling is actually working better than the drugs ever did!"

You, too, can combine the tuning practices in this section with good eating and daily exercise for optimal health and well-being. While the tips below may seem like a beautiful daily practice, you may find it challenging to dedicate a few hours in the morning and evening to incorporate them.

My suggestion is to do your best in terms of how much you can do during the week. Remember, even if you adopt a couple of tuning practices, that in itself is good to kick start the healing or wellness process. Furthermore, you can try to bring in most of the practices during holidays or weekends, when more time is available.

Follow this routine to incorporate all of the aforementioned suggestions into your day:

- *5:00 a.m.: After waking up, drink a glass of warm water on an empty stomach. Cleanse your tongue with a scraper, and then rinse your mouth with water. Now, take one teaspoon of any suitable oil and complete the oil pulling for two to five minutes. Spit out the oil and rinse your mouth with water.*

- *5:15 a.m.: Select a bitter twig or root and chew on it until it forms the bristles. Use the bristles to brush the teeth and clean the gums.*

- *5:30 a.m.: Use the neti pot for nasal cleansing.*

- *5:45 a.m.: Pour some massage oil (containing essential oils) onto your palm, and massage your scalp, eyes, ears, nose, abdomen, back, hips, legs, top, and bottom of your feet. Use circular strokes on the joints, and long, repetitive strokes on your limbs and bony areas. Leave the oil on the body until you are ready to take a shower.*

- *6:00 a.m.: While your body is soaking in the oil, focus on the eyes. Splash cool water into your eyes three to five times. Gently dry your eyes with a cloth towel. Now, exercise your eyes by moving them right and left, upward and downward, and clockwise and counterclockwise. Following this, repeat the palm cupping procedure twice.*

- *6:15 a.m.: Give yourself an intraocular massage. Use one of the two options from the tuning and maintenance suggestions for the eye.*
- *6:30 a.m.: Perform karna mastiska yoga at least nine times while facing the rising sun. This further enhances the absorption of the oil through the sense organs.*
- *6:45 a.m.: Step out and go for a short walk and be mindful of the sounds of nature. Inhale and exhale, and if you find that your mind has wandered, simply bring it back to the sounds of nature.*
- *7:30 a.m.: Take a shower and gently massage every part of the body with warm water.*
- *8:00 a.m.: By the time you have finished some of your sensory therapies as well as your walk, it is time to eat breakfast (especially if you had your previous night meal by 7:00 p.m. since you have fasted your body and brain for nearly twelve hours).*

Assuming you ate dinner by 7:00 p.m., follow these routines before going to bed:

- *8:00 p.m.: Repeat the trataka or lamp gazing sequence two times. See the tuning and maintenance section for the eyes for a detailed description.*
- *8:15 p.m.: Give yourself an intraocular massage.*

- *8:30 p.m.: Use nasya therapy to cleanse your nose.*
- *8:45 p.m.: Using the fluid dropper, oleate your ear. See the tuning and maintenance section for the ears for greater detail.*
- *9:00 p.m.: Pour some massage oil on your palm and massage your temples, eyes, and the bottom of your feet. You may leave the oil on your body before going to bed. (Note: If you are concerned about soiling the sheets, wear loose cotton socks and cover your feet.)*

Remember, for optimal wellness, you will want to combine tuning practices with a regular exercise regimen and a healthy, high-prana diet (mentioned in the previous chapters) and good living practices mentioned in the later chapters.

PART II

GOOD MENTAL PRACTICES

More than just Good Physical Practices, it is imperative to include Good Mental Practices into your life to keep your mind tuned and sharp. When I use the word "mind," I am referring to the brain, and I will use these terms interchangeably since mental practice includes the skills needed to strengthen the brain and nervous system—the conduits through which energy and information flow.

GOOD MENTAL PRACTICES are about reinforcing the structural and functional aspects of the brain, and this can be achieved through the following:

CHAPTER 4: SCULPTING THE BRAIN

Neuroplasticity is the key to your brain's resilience and strength. Mental training exercises for sculpting the brain are critical in keeping you mentally sharp, confident, and focused.

CHAPTER 5: SLEEP – A PILLAR OF LIFE

Because sleep plays a vital role in good health and wellness, this chapter delves into the necessary practices to develop healthy sleeping habits. Quality sleep strengthens your emotions, mind, and physical health as well as improving your overall quality of life.

CHAPTER 6: SELFLESS SERVICE

Engaging in acts of selfless service reinforces both the mind and body. People who incorporate selfless service into their daily lives strengthen their ability to resist the ego's impulses and instead achieve greater fulfillment and happiness. By performing selfless service, you will be inspired to do the right thing, while being less impulsive and/or driven to act on knee-jerk or selfish urges.

CHAPTER 4

SCULPTING THE BRAIN

"If you do not use a muscle, or any part of the body, it tends to become atrophic. So is the case with the brain. The more you use it, the better it becomes."

SHAKUNTALA DEVI

Psychologists think of the "mind" as the part of us that regulates our energy and information flow. Throughout this book, I will refer to the mind as the organic, functional nature of the mind (a.k.a., the brain), including its numerous neural networks. In other words, when I refer to the mind, think of the brain and the information flow through its associated nerves.

According to Ayurveda and Yoga texts, disease first begins with the emotions, then spreads to the mind, and (when left unchecked) later appears in the body in the form of specific symptoms. Fortunately, modern science now acknowledges and accepts that there is a powerful mind-body connection, and this has helped us better understand how intellectual, mental, social, and behavioral factors influence health outcomes and well-being.[58]

To maintain mental fitness, then, it is imperative to keep the brain in a healthy state through mentally stimulating tasks. Brain fitness, mental fitness, and mental exercise all mean the same thing. These tasks help you become more alert, sensible, and rational by stimulating new neural connections. Keeping the brain sharp can help prevent age-associated memory decline and cognitive loss. And because of the mind-body-emotions nexus, it is not surprising that those who possess a higher level of mental agility also tend to be physically healthy and live a high-quality, harmonious life.[59]

Research findings indicate that humans actually build and rebuild brain cells throughout their lives.[60] In fact, if you engage in a learning environment that maintains, builds, and remodels your neural network connectivity, this will also trigger the production of nerve growth factors that stimulate new neural connections. This active growth in the brain is termed "neuroplasticity," and it refers to the capacity of the brain to mold and rewire itself through stimulating and challenging learning and experiences. Any challenging or stimulating mental exercise that increases neuroplasticity also fosters brain strength and resilience.[61]

Envision neuroplasticity as a process that's similar to walking along trails in the forest. If you've ever taken a walk in the woods, you have probably noticed that frequent use causes the trail to get broader and wider. Over time, these trails appear more and more obvious as they become well established. In the same way, your brain is constantly changing, sculpting, and rewiring itself in response to new experiences and learning.[62] As these new neuronal branches get stronger, they too become well established and permanent.[63]

Neuroplasticity is the reason stroke patients can relearn skills after brain damage, as the healthy part of the brain assumes the job of a damaged part. And just as it is with stroke patients, so it is with our aging brains, where unfavorable changes take place. However, we can ward off some of these changes through a high prana diet, regular exercise, tuning of the body, and by engaging in as many brain-stimulating exercises as possible.[64]

Unlike other systemic areas in our bodies, the brain is created with a finite number of cells and has a limited capacity for regeneration. As a result, certain areas of the brain shrink in size as we age, including the prefrontal cortex and the hippocampus. Blood flow to the brain also reduces with age because the arteries shrink, and there is a reduction in the growth of new capillaries.

Structures called plaques and tangles—a subset of poorly formed proteins—accumulate inside and outside of the brain to disrupt the communication network between neurons and provoke the inflammatory process. If this inflammation goes unchecked, it can elicit several brain disorders. And if that isn't bad enough, aging also triggers the production of free radicals—byproducts of chemical processes in the cell. These free radicals have a tendency to interact with cellular structures, trigger their destruction, and exacerbate the inflammatory process.

Together with changes in the brain's physical structure, its mental capacity and function also change with age. Generally, people complain about an inability to learn new things, retrieve information, and experience challenges with the latest technological aids. They will also perform poorly on complex tasks of attention, learning, and memory. That's because the functions attributed to the cortex and hippocampus (learning, memory acquisition, recall, planning, cognitive behavior, personality, social behavior, and decision-making) all become compromised with each passing year.

While there is a general decline in physical structure and mental abilities, a mentally active person's brain will appear like a dense forest of thickly branched neural connectivity, even in older people.[65] Brain fitness that promotes connectivity can occur in a variety of ways. Research studies find that mental exercises can delay the onset of neurodegenerative diseases, cancer, and other stress-associated disorders. These brain-strengthening activities include: solving complex equations and puzzles, reading, visual-spatial learning, exposure to new experiences, memorizing passages and texts, and recalling correctly whatever is memorized.[66]

The London taxi cab study is a perfect example of the brain's neuroplasticity response to mental challenges. London taxi drivers undergo four years of exhaustive training, including memorizing all of London's streets, secondary roads, by-lanes, and alleys. Then, the drivers-in-training appear for a unique intellectual, psychological, and physical examination that is considered the hardest taxi test of any kind in the world.[67]

In contrast to bus drivers—whose driving routes are well established and unchanging—London taxi drivers' extensive training allows them to navigate effortlessly to thousands of places within the city, demonstrating powerful spatial expertise. Constantly learning new routes in the city and reorganizing those routes is a mental exercise that forces the cab drivers' brains to transform and create new neural connections. Over time, this extensive neural branching changes the structure and size of the brain.[68]

In the United States, automobiles have steering wheels on the left side, while the driver travels on the right side of the road. In contrast, the United States Postal Service jeeps are right-hand-driven vehicles, allowing the carrier to drop off mail in the mailboxes that are located on the right side of the road. Postal carriers constantly switch between their private left-hand-drive vehicles and the right-hand-drive postal jeeps, thereby continually challenging their brains. It is my belief that the incidence of Alzheimer's and dementia may be relatively low among United States postal carriers, although this needs to be tested through a proper research study. Furthermore, if the US postal drivers were to combine their daily postal duties with good eating practices, physical exercise, regular tuning of their senses, and other good practices mentioned in later chapters, it follows that they will have optimal health and wellness.

However, you don't need to be a postal carrier to challenge your brain throughout your lifetime. By learning new things, trying out different hobbies and interests, and constantly engaging in mentally stimulating activities, you too can keep your brain strong. The mental fitness exercises I suggest throughout the rest of this chapter are ones that you can perform in a variety of settings to improve your memory, attention, and visual-spatial skills.

Memory

Our memory is the brain's filing system. It stores everything we have learned and continue to learn. Certain areas of the brain lay down the memory, while other areas are involved in storage and memory retrieval.

During intense learning, neurons from these different areas wire up with one other and communicate through thousands of connections. Memories get consolidated when these connections are strengthened.

The following activities will strengthen your memory by boosting the level of brain chemicals that are responsible for memory, storage, consolidation, and retrieval: reading, learning by rote, reasoning, mental calculation, memorizing the lyrics of a new song or street signs in a new area, learning a new language, and completing crossword and math puzzles.

Here are some easy ways to get started:

AIRPORT MEMORY GAME

The next time you board a plane, recall your gate number, as well as the flight number and destination of the flight that preceded yours. After you reach your destination, try recalling this information.

PARKING LOT MEMORIES

After parking your car at the shopping mall, observe the color, make, and model of the car parked on your left and the car parked on your right. Write down the information and tuck it away until later. After completing your shopping (and before you return to your car), recall the specifics of those two cars. Review your notes to verify your answers.

PARAPHERNALIA GAME

Ask your spouse or friend to arrange a variety of kitchen items on a serving tray. Give yourself sixty seconds to survey the utensils, measuring cups, etc. Now, cover the tray with a cloth and try to recall all the items. Note the time it takes you to remember as much as you can. Repeat this memory test with a new set of items to practice again and track your improvement.

Attention

Attention and memory go hand-hand. Attention is necessary to consolidate memories, maintain concentration, focus on a task, and complete multiple tasks in a timely manner. Our power of choice can also affect our attention since that which receives the greatest attention from us will remain in our memory, while things we pay little attention to will be forgotten.[69]

One way to improve attention is by simply changing your daily routines and habits. This forces your brain to remain active, as well as sprout new neural branches and networks. New experiences also build new connections and set us on the path to mental fitness. Here are a couple more ways to improve your attention and challenge your brain:

GOAL GAME

Think about a specific task (reading, writing, cooking, etc.) that you would like to accomplish. Set a timer for a brief period of time (for example, twenty minutes). As you engage in the task, remain attentive as long as you can without getting distracted until the timer goes off. When the timer beeps, attempt to recall each step you took during the task, and ask yourself: *Was I fully attentive to the task? How often was I distracted?*

NEW ROUTE MEMORY

If you typically drive the same way to work, try taking a completely different route to your workplace without the use of the GPS. After you reach your destination, recall the names of all the streets that you used.

Visual-Spatial Awareness

Visual-spatial awareness involves seeing, organizing, remembering, and differentiating objects of attention. It is about recognizing symbols, images or words, and understanding that they differ from one another. It involves discrimination between objects of different sizes, shapes, and colors. It also includes the ability to realize when certain parts of an object are visible (or not).

Those who face visual-spatial challenges have difficulty reading, recognizing, or appreciating maps, diagrams, pictures, layouts, or schedules. Visual-spatial impairment is often an early symptom of a neurological condition that involves memory.[70]

Challenge your brain with the following tasks to improve your own visual-spatial awareness:

ROOM AWARENESS

The next time you are in the lobby of a hotel, doctor's office, or another place of business, look around and notice all the objects in the room. Choose five items to remember, as well as their location in the room. After exiting the building, try to remember each item and the location. Then, challenge yourself to remember these details an hour later (and again after twenty-four hours).

OBJECT AWARENESS

Look around a room in your home and jot down at least five rectangular objects and five red objects. Flip the list over and exit the room. Now, try to remember all the rectangular and red objects. Challenge yourself to remember these objects an hour later and again the next day. Repeat this exercise once a day and challenge your brain by noting two or more different shapes and several colored objects simultaneously.

Flexibility

This is the ability to transition between multiple concepts simultaneously, as well as react and respond to changing goals, new situations, or novel environmental stimuli. The faster a person can switch from a concept, goal, or stimulus to another, the greater mental flexibility they possess. Many times, responses have become a habit, and people who are unable to transition between multiple concepts simultaneously or cannot break their habitual thought patterns are said to be in a state of "cognitive rigidity."

To keep your brain flexible, try the tasks below:

HAND-SWITCHING

If you prefer using one hand over the other, start performing tasks with your non-dominant hand. I use my right hand for most chores, so I have now started training my brain by using my left hand for eating or computer work. While this transition was fairly smooth for me, I found using the computer mouse with the left hand to be challenging. Check it out and see if you can develop proficiency using your non-dominant hand.

NEW HOBBIES OR INTERESTS

Try something new that you've always wanted to explore. For example, learn a musical instrument or new language to sustain mental flexibility.

Your Brain and the Five Senses

The five sense organs, with their corresponding senses (i.e., sound, touch, sight, taste, and smell) have a close association with the brain and its cognitive function. For this reason, I call these feeder pathways to the brain. As a result, any structural or functional loss of the senses will also have an impact on brain structure and function, resulting in cognitive failure.[71] Unhealthy impressions drawn through the five senses may also have an adverse effect on the structure and function of the brain, snowballing into the physical body and manifesting as gross symptoms, pain, and suffering.[72]

The information that follows will detail exactly why proper care for your sense organs and keeping your senses sharp are some of the best ways to maintain brain health:

BRAIN AND EARS

While you might think of brain function and hearing as two independent events, recent research reports clearly show that both cognitive impairment and hearing loss are age-associated degenerative events and that there is a close association between auditory loss and declining cognition with age.[73] A decline in one of these areas negatively influences the other. Since cognitive decline worsens as hearing becomes increasingly impaired, researchers believe that auditory loss may precede cognitive dysfunction. However, restoring hearing function may improve or at least delay cognitive decline.[74] In addition to the recommendations in Chapter 3, speech and music therapy are possible interventions to improve hearing and, thereby, cognition.

BRAIN AND SKIN

If you've ever had a massage, then you know how calm and relaxed you feel after treatment. While this type of therapy certainly benefits the body, I believe that keeping your skin healthy benefits your brain as well. Cause and effect can be difficult to ascertain, yet research suggests that emotional upheavals can trigger certain skin conditions, pointing to the bond between skin and mind (the brain). With such a deeply rooted connection, it is not surprising to note that the medical subspecialty called psychodermatology primarily treats skin disorders using psychological and psychiatric techniques.[75]

The brain-skin connection is established early with the formation of the embryo. The ectoderm, one of the three primordial structures in the young embryo, separates to form the brain and skin. Knowing that the brain and skin originate from the same primordial lineage, it is not far-fetched to think that anything that affects the brain may affect the skin, and vice-versa—and research supports this idea. The skin reacts to stress-induced changes in the brain by activating the body's defense systems, and mental stress negatively impacts skin structure and function.[76]

To prove that a link indeed exists between the brain and skin, I embarked on a project that involved taking normal mouse skin and brain tissue, breaking them apart, and making a cellular extract and analyzing the proteins from each one. If there were an authentic brain-skin connection, it would be reflected in both the brain and skin samples possessing similar proteins. Through this study, we discovered that nearly half a dozen brain proteins were present in the skin extract as well, thus reinforcing the brain-skin link.

Researchers are now searching for molecules that mediate the brain-skin connection, with the hope that any issues in the brain could be foreseen by examining the skin and using it as a conduit to deliver drugs to the brain. However, until researchers have developed these new therapies, I suggest that you incorporate the various home-based therapies for the skin, as described in Chapter 3.

BRAIN AND EYES

Like your other sense organs, the eyes have a direct connection to the brain, and research provides a link between poor vision and cognitive decline. Because it appears that age-associated loss in vision likely drives cognitive decline, protecting one's vision may help prevent cognitive deterioration.[77] Again, paying attention to the various home-based therapies for eyes, as described in Chapter 3, will benefit both vision and the brain.

BRAIN, TONGUE, AND NOSE

An inability to identify smell or taste precedes the clinical manifestation of several neurodegenerative and neuropsychiatric diseases, highlighting the roles of taste and smell as markers for early interventions. Additionally, the unanimous opinion among researchers is that oral health is also related to brain health. Although there is no clear causal relationship between the two, people with poor oral health tend to have memory issues. Poor oral hygiene triggers periodontitis, which is characterized by redness, swelling, and bleeding of the gums. The bacteria that set off this inflammatory condition not only attack the bones and tissues in the mouth but also invade the brain through the bloodstream, resulting in brain-related illness, including stroke and Alzheimer's disease.[78]

Hyposmia is the technical term to indicate a reduced ability to smell and to detect odors, while anosmia is a condition in which a person cannot detect any odors at all. Ayurvedic medicine has long recognized the nexus between the nose, smell sensation, and brain structure and function. As mentioned earlier, it is believed that a loss of sense of smell, deficits in other senses, and metabolic disturbances may be a symptom that later manifests as age-associated neurodegenerative diseases.[79] Recent research confirms that in neurological diseases like epilepsy, Alzheimer's, and Parkinson's, losing one's sense of smell is a common yet unnoticed symptom that may occur several years prior to the actual neurological diagnosis.[80]

The oral cavity (mouth) and nose serve as the gateway to the brain, owing to the absence of an effective barrier between these regions and the brain. While this serves as a good delivery route for drugs to reach the brain directly, it can be risky as well—especially if someone does not maintain good nasal and oral hygiene practices. The remote idea that microbes trigger Alzheimer's disease (AD) is now gaining traction among the scientific community.

Neuroscientists now believe that poor nasal and oral hygiene practices give certain pathogens direct access to the brain and contribute to symptoms, including memory loss and cognitive decline. Thus, to keep the brain healthy and functional, it is imperative that we maintain good oral and nasal hygiene practices. Check the activities listed in *Tips from the GLP Toolbox in* Chapter 3, to keep the nose and oral cavity (mouth) strong and healthy.

Other Brain Connections

In addition to the five senses, other systemic organs maintain a close connection with the brain. Keeping these organs happy and healthy is akin to keeping the brain healthy and resilient.

BRAIN-BODY NEXUS

Engaging in regular physical exercise leads to structural changes in the brain that improve memory and cognition. Physical exercise increases nerve branching and nerve-to-nerve communication, especially in the memory centers of the brain.[81]

Have you ever felt so tired at the end of a workday that your brain refuses to function smoothly? To keep your brain sharp, it's best to hit the gym instead of the couch after a long workday. I sometimes have to force myself to work out after a long day, but once I get to the gym, it's so invigorating and rewarding that I'm always glad I went, and this keeps me in a high prana state.

How does physical exercise activate these brain changes? Neuroscientists believe that physical exercises trigger increased blood flow to the brain, which brings with it more oxygen and other vital nutrients. However, a combination of age and poor health practices results in a decline in the volume of the blood flow into the brain. This, in turn, decreases the hemoglobin, sugar and oxygen content to the brain that may result in age-associated cognitive and mental problems.[82]

According to yoga texts, any physical posture that involves hanging upside down (head-down position) will lead to increased blood circulation to the brain. A good supply of blood to the brain will reduce and remove toxic proteins, support the regeneration of brain neural networks, strengthen the blood vessels that supply the brain, and repair any damage that has already occurred, thereby enhancing cognition.[83]

Inverted yoga postures are a great routine to add to your daily list of exercises. They will improve blood flow to the brain, thereby reducing the risk of age-associated neurodegenerative conditions. If you are a beginner (or not familiar with these poses), it is best to seek out instruction from a qualified yoga teacher. You can also consider using an inversion table, which is primarily used by chiropractors to stretch the spine (spinal traction) in an attempt to relieve back pain. Be sure to consult your physician if you plan to use the inversion table since it could be risky for anyone with high blood pressure, heart disease, glaucoma, or severe back issues.

In addition to warding off cognitive decline, physical exercises also help maintain optimal blood pressure, control diabetes, and lower cholesterol levels, all of which are potential mental health risk factors.[84] In addition, physical exercise boosts the production of a chemical called brain-derived neurotrophic factor (BDNF).

BDNF supports the survival of existing neurons, improves nerve-to-nerve connectivity, stimulates new nerve branching, and triggers the growth and differentiation of new neurons.[85] The higher the BDNF levels in the brain, the stronger the neuron and nerve-to-nerve communication, thereby morphing the brain into greater resiliency. This may explain the cognitive improvements associated with physical exercise.[86]

Yet another brain-body link is the one between the brain and digestion. If you recall from Chapter 1, I suggested the need for a minimum twelve-hour fast between two meals. This fasting window allows the brain cells to switch from glucose to fat digestion, leading to the release of good fats with neuroprotective properties. Interestingly, physical exercise triggers the production of these same good fats. What's more, one of the functions of these good fats is to boost the production of BDNF, which also supports nerve growth. Thus, multiple, overlapping pathways are stimulated by physical exercise, fasting, and mindful eating—which converge on the BDNF pathway to benefit the brain and the body.

The concept of "use it or lose it" applies not only to your body but also to the nerve pathways and connections in our brains. Efficient communication between your brain's neurons improves cognition, helping you reap the benefits of a sharper mind and healthier body for years to come. Researchers are not surprised to observe that people who exercise their brains and bodies lead longer, higher quality, and healthier lives.[87]

BRAIN-BONE NEXUS

The skeletal system, which is comprised of all your bones and joints, provides structural support to the body. Various cells, proteins, and minerals make up the skeletal system, which acts as a scaffold, providing support and protection to the softer tissues of the body. Until recently, it was assumed that the skeletal system was an inert, calcified structure that only provided a framework to prevent the body from collapsing. Thanks to groundbreaking work, we now know that there's more to the bones than just the support structure and it involves the brain.[88]

Neuroscientists have discovered a new link between brain and bone, and the message is that brain health is linked closely to bone health. The brain and bone communicate closely with each other. The signals from the brain that control digestion, satiety, appetite, obesity, and energy also alter bone density. Many neurochemicals that were previously thought to be involved in nerve-to-nerve communication in the brain are now shown to play a major role in nerve-to-bone signaling, as well as bone-to-bone signaling. Evidence also suggests that the same neural mechanism underlying brain modulation is responsible for bone remodeling (a physiological process that involves reshaping or replacing damaged bone by new bone tissue, following injuries or micro-damage that occurs during normal activity), healing of fractures, and even bone development.[89]

As we age, our skeletal system degenerates, resulting in reduced bone mass. Additionally, aging is associated with declining memory, cognitive loss, and emotional turbulence. Recent research studies have suggested that the age-associated degenerative events in the physical body, memory decline, and emotions may all be interconnected. For example, scientists have shown that negative emotions can affect bone density.[90] Chronic depression sets off nerve signals and the release of certain neurochemicals that have crippling effects on bone density and remodeling, suggesting that any healing modalities should involve both the brain and the bone. Interestingly, physical exercise does just that. It strengthens the bone and skeletal system, while also preventing age-associated cognitive losses.[91]

Research studies show that physical exercise stimulates and remodels bone growth, improves bone density, improves the mood, stimulates new neural cell growth, and triggers branching of nerves.[92] This provides a compelling reason to engage in regular physical exercise to stay healthy, both physically and mentally.

BRAIN-COLON NEXUS

I often have students or patients complaining about unexplained headaches or pain in the lower back, hips, or knees. Most of them also describe having poor bowel movements (e.g., skipping for two or more days). In the Ayurveda system of medicine, there is a close link between the brain and colon. This realization helps people in the Ayurveda community take steps to address their colon and normalize their bowel movements. Meanwhile, people who are unaware of Ayurveda wisdom continue to complain about the unexplained headaches or joint aches without realizing that to address the pain, they would need to correct their diet, normalize the gut, and stabilize colon function.[93]

If you eat three nourishing, high-prana meals daily, you will become regular and rarely skip a day. In contrast, low prana foods prevent colonic movement, leading to constipation. Chronic constipation leads to a myriad of colon diseases, including diverticular disease, hemorrhoids, anal fissures, rectal prolapse, and colorectal cancer. Ayurveda takes this one step further, considering constipation to be a prelude to other problems affecting the skeletal and nervous systems. Ayurveda suggests that a well-functioning colon supports brain, bones, spine, joints, and ligaments, while a poorly functioning colon can create chronic issues in any or all of the above-mentioned areas. It is my belief that chronic constipation and a host of other colon disorders arise primarily from a highly processed, low-prana diet that is devoid of fiber and water.

In contrast to Ayurveda recommendations, the western diet primarily consists of heavily processed grains, refined sugars and oils, fatty meats, and copious amounts of salt. This low prana diet is devoid of fiber and water, resulting in harmful effects on health, especially colonic health. In the United States alone, approximately 20 percent of the population suffers from constipation, and the cost of treating constipation is nearly $821 million a year.[94]

If you notice a pattern of missed bowel movements, make sure you are eating a high-prana diet. And the next time you have a migraine, chronic low back pain, knee issues, or unexplained joint pain, ask yourself when you had your last bowel movement; there may a direct link. Although you may be enjoying the culinary pleasures of an affluent lifestyle, chronic constipation suggests that you are occupying the bottommost rung of the good health and wellness ladder.

According to modern science, our body has a second brain: the colon. In fact, scientists use the term "colon intelligence," because the colon can function without instructions from the brain.[95] The millions of neurons in the colonic tract coordinate the muscle contractions for fecal waste to exit out at a steady pace and in the right direction. The neuronal firing pattern in the colon follows a rhythmic pattern similar to brain waves and helps to eliminate the fecal material. The rhythmic wave pattern is so striking and similar that researchers believe that, in addition to removing waste, the colon also influences our emotions. Surely, acute or chronic mental stress leads to chronic constipation and vice-versa, as poor bowel movements prompt depression and mental illness.[96] Thus, mental stress and constipation lead a person down a spiral of despair, depression, or general angst.[97]

BRAIN-GUT NEXUS

The body of evidence linking healthy eating and the gut to the brain is growing rapidly. Physically speaking, poor digestion leads to many gut problems, including, but not limited to, bloating, diarrhea, acidity, GERD, and ulcers. When the gut malfunctions, every other body part—including the brain goes haywire.[98] Having gut issues is neither normal nor healthy. A healthy digestive system is more important than we believe, as it is home to nearly 100 million neurons and host to hundreds of neurochemicals that regulate the fine balance between the gut and brain.

Whether you realize it or not, you have most likely had experiences where the brain affects your gut. Think back to those times you've felt that strange, unexplained sensation in your stomach before taking an exam or appearing for an interview. This is an example of your brain and gut communicating with one another.[99] The reverse is also true: Whenever you experience stomach pain, discomfort, nausea, bloating, or acidity, it is the gut communicating to the brain that something is amiss with the food you recently ate.

The gut is a reservoir of beneficial bacteria—the microbiome essential to overall health. This microbiome works closely with the body's immune (defense) system, nutrient absorption, body weight regulation, blood glucose control, insulin sensitivity, and the production of several neurochemicals and neurohormones.[100] The gut directly affects brain function, emotions, and cognitive health—while diet, lifestyle, and other age-related changes affect the microbiome and among the chief causes of most chronic conditions, inflammatory diseases, and neurological disease.[101] Following the suggestions for Good Physical Practices in Part 1 will not only support a healthy community of gut bacteria but also sustain optimal brain health throughout your life.

Tips from the GLP Toolbox for Brain Sculpting

Try these additional suggestions to strengthen your brain, as well as your body and sense organs:

- *If you are stuck in traffic, instead of cursing at the people and cars around you, engage in mental exercises instead. For example, observe license plates' designs and state slogans, as well as car colors and makes. Try to memorize these details and recall them later that day.*

- *Learn a new language to strengthen neural connections.*
- *During your free time, solve puzzles like word searches, crosswords, Sudoku, and logic puzzles. If you are with a group of people, engage in intelligent card games such as bridge or blackjack, as these games require reasoning, logic, and concentration, along with social interaction.*
- *Memorize complicated verses from religious books or other texts. Several research studies have now demonstrated that memorizing verses, texts, lyrics, or mantras increases the size of the brain regions associated with cognitive function, including memory and thinking.*
- *Learn to play a musical instrument. This requires learning and memorizing new notes, rhythm, beats, etc., all of which are wonderful cognitive exercises. Wind instruments, in particular, promote diaphragmatic (belly) breathing and require powerful airflow. Playing a wind instrument actually engages the mind, abdominal muscles, lungs, and heart—a perfect example of exercising the brain and body.*

Reminder: For optimal results, continue to integrate the practices from all previous and future chapters into your daily routine. The more practices you can include in your life, the more results you will see!

CHAPTER 5

SLEEP – A PILLAR OF LIFE

"Each night, when I go to sleep, I die. And the next morning, when I wake up, I am reborn."

MAHATMA GANDHI

According to Ayurveda philosophy, sleep is one of the three main pillars of life. It endows the body and brain with strength and healthy growth that continues throughout one's lifespan, provided he or she does not indulge in activities that result in sleeplessness or insomnia. And although many people pay attention to diet and physical exercise, they might ignore the fact that good sleep contributes to good health as well and sleep deficiencies can cause acute and chronic health problems.[102]

To reach our full potential, we must cultivate a healthy sleeping practice since it affects the way we think, react, work, or learn. A good night of sleep enhances positive feelings and plays a direct role in how full, energetic, and successful our lives can be. Proper sleep and rest also influence emotions, nourishment, emaciation, strength, weakness, virility, knowledge, life, and even our mortality.

According to the *Harvard Women's Health Watch*, sleep is a necessity for several reasons:[103]

- *The body utilizes sleep to repair itself of any damage sustained during the waking hours.*
- *Sleep regulates the appetite by optimizing the levels of hormones that play a role in hunger and satiety. Sleep deprivation can, therefore, trigger weight gain.*
- *Sleep helps the brain sustain memory consolidation, preserve new information, and enhance cognition.*
- *People who have good sleep habits perform better on various tasks and tests.*

- *Sleep deprivation contributes to emotional disturbances, accidents, falls, and traffic mishaps.*
- *Sleep disorders can cause hypertension and an irregular heartbeat.*
- *Sleep deprivation weakens the immune system, making you more susceptible to degenerative diseases or infections. In contrast, good quality sleep contributes to a healthy immune system, helping you to thrive.*

Sleep researchers have discovered that having good, sound sleep quality allows the brain to clear out harmful toxins, thereby reducing the risk of several brain diseases. During good quality sleep, there is a dramatic increase in the flow of cerebrospinal fluid in the brain, draining away waste proteins that build up during the day.[104] This cleansing process reduces the risk of age-associated dementia or dementia due to Alzheimer's disease because the waste proteins that are being washed away are toxic to brain cells. This may explain why it is hard to think clearly after experiencing a sleepless night and why prolonged lack of sleep is damaging to health.[105]

Sleep also helps us to erase some of the extraneous things we learn each day. Because learning requires new neuronal connections, this process helps neurons to communicate with other neighboring neurons quickly and efficiently. These new branches store memories of events, tasks, and impressions that we draw daily through our five senses. When these branches grow wildly from experiential learning, our neuronal circuits actually get "noisy" from all of the continuous electrical activity. While some of the information we receive each day is helpful and important, some of it is either useless or redundant and does not need to be stored, as it takes up too much "brain space."

The brain tries to avoid storing all of the information that we encounter on a day to day basis, especially the bad, unpleasant, sad, and negative events. Your brain's memory center does not want to store these negative thoughts and experiences. For example, if your lunch order got delayed, or you disappointed friends by missing an important appointment, you've created unnecessary "brain noise" that needs to be erased. When we sleep soundly, the brain discards all of this unnecessary noise and consolidates just the relevant signals. Good quality sleep activates the pruning machinery to trim the excess neuronal branches formed from some of the recent events in your life.

Unfortunately, the pruning of irrelevant experiences and the consolidation of memories is less efficient in people with sleep issues, resulting in more neuronal noise and fuzzy memories. Over time, these disharmonious memories accumulate in the brain, eventually harming the individual.[106]

In addition to contributing to psychological health and well being, proper sleep serves as an antidote to fear, because specific fear memories are wiped out during sound sleep. In contrast, poor sleep blocks the proper repair of the brain. Sleep deprivation/disturbance is a major source of stress among adults, and the consequences include severe mood disturbances, depression, and emotional upheaval. Studies show that lack of sleep (or discontinuous sleep during the night) can be harmful to the brain, triggering dementia and increasing the risk of other neurodegenerative conditions.[107]

Sadly, we live in a world of unhealthy sleepers.[108] Statistical studies on insomnia and poor quality sleep confirm this. Between 40 and 60 percent of people over the age of sixty suffer from insomnia, with women twice as likely to suffer as men. To promote better sleep, the sleep-aid industry has created a slew of sleep aids, pills, drugs, and devices to diagnose and treat sleep disorders, including sleep apnea and insomnia.

In 2016, when the rest of the world accounted for 8 percent of the world's sleep aid market, the United States alone accounted for a whopping 65 percent of the total share and world revenues in the global sleep aid market was $69.5 billion in 2017, and analysts say the sleep-aid industry will generate $100 billion by 2023. Clearly, insomnia is a major health issue, and as a result, more and more people are seeking sleep aids for relief.[109]

Sleep aids claim to help improve the quality of sleep by reducing the time required to fall asleep and increasing the duration of quality sleep. While mattresses and pillows make up the largest part of the sleeping aid market, the use of sleeping pills is also common, with about 10 to 20 percent of the global population currently using pills for relief from insomnia and other sleep disorders. The United States' share of more than 48 percent represents the largest market for sleeping pills globally.[110]

Interestingly and of major concern is the fact that sleeping pills are no longer specific to the elderly, as indicated by an exponential rise in the number of people between the ages of twenty and forty-five who claim to use sleeping pills regularly. Unfortunately, sleeping pills may not be a panacea, they only help people fall asleep eight to twenty minutes faster and increase total sleep time by about twenty to thirty minutes.[111] Thus, the risks associated with sleeping pills outweigh the benefits, especially considering the immense harm these sleeping pills can cause to a person,[112] including:

- *Constipation or diarrhea*
- *Addiction*
- *Poor appetite, bloating, and other digestive issues*
- *Burning or tingling in the hands, arms, feet, or legs*

- *Dizziness and/or difficulty keeping balance*
- *Drowsiness, lethargy, and unexplained pains*
- *Dryness*

There is quite a price to pay if you are experiencing sleep problems. According to experts, teenagers need eight to ten hours of sleep each night, young adults and adults need seven to nine hours, and older adults need seven to eight hours. And it's not just getting a certain number of hours that's vital; the time you go to bed and how often you wake up throughout the night are key factors, too. Sleep researchers have compared interrupted sleep (the kind where you go to bed at the normal time but constantly wake up every few hours) and abbreviated sleep (the kind where you go to bed very late in the night and get two to four hours of uninterrupted sleep). Studies have found that both are unhealthy to the body and mind, but among the two, interrupted sleep is unhealthier than abbreviated sleep.[113]

Those who report interrupted sleep regularly experience a significant decline in positive moods, coupled with an increase in negative emotions. Furthermore, if the interrupted sleep is chronic, it impairs their ability to recover or stabilize positive emotions. Therefore, we need to pay attention to not just the quantity or quality of sleep but also the combination of our sleep and moods.[114]

Lost sleep is another issue. In fact, losing one or more hours of sleep can place you into serious sleep debt. Researchers believe those with chronic sleep debt have a hard time catching up on lost sleep hours, increasing the likelihood of sleep deprivation symptoms. Yes, additional hours of sleep may provide some benefits, like being less groggy and more alert, but it will not truly make up for the lost sleep hours. In fact, you would actually need four days of good quality sleep to overcome one hour of sleep debt.[115] Since most people get less sleep than what is normally recommended, sleep debt accumulates with time and raises the risk for several chronic health problems, affecting how well you think, react, work, and learn.

In several research studies, mindfulness and meditation were shown to be powerful interventions to improve sleep quality and reduce fatigue. Even those experiencing abbreviated sleep but who practiced mindfulness and meditation felt more refreshed after waking up, felt less distressed about insomnia, and were better able to cope with sleeplessness. Therefore, a yoga program consisting of breathing exercises, yoga postures (asanas), and meditation is a useful intervention for improving sleep quality and reducing sleep medication.[116] Furthermore, listening to soft music or sounds of nature (rain forest, the rustling of leaves, temple bells, or water flowing down the rocks, etc.) triggers the relaxation response and reduces the body's natural fight-or-flight response that may also assist with the sleep.[117]

Follow the reminders below to begin improving your sleep quality, naturally without resorting to sleeping aids:

DIET

Follow the recommendations from Chapter 1, by eating healthy, freshly prepared high-prana foods like fruit, vegetables, pulses, and whole grains. At the same time, avoid low-prana foods. Remember that the farther the food is from its natural state, the less prana it possesses. Also, keep in mind the following:

- *Avoid highly-processed foods, fast foods, frozen foods, ready-to-eat foods, canned/tinned foods, deep-fried foods, and stale foods especially at night, as they can increase brain activity, making it more difficult to get good quality sleep.*

- *Acidic, highly fermented, or spicy foods, meat (especially red meat), and foods high in caffeine, sugar, and alcohol all suppress sleep and should be avoided, especially at night. Say no to coffee, soda, lattes, or any stimulating beverages as well. If you have chronic sleep issues, consider cutting off the consumption of these beverages after lunch or eliminate them completely. Avoiding these foods and beverages improves the chances of achieving restorative sleep.*

- *If you are stressed or fatigued, quieten your body and mind before eating a meal with a few gentle yoga stretches, deep breathing, or a few minutes of meditation. A short walk can work wonders, too!*

- *Our digestive system is endowed with an internal clock that is influenced by the time of the day. Thus, having your dinner by 7.00 p.m. not only prevents digestive related problems but also ensures good sleep.*

- *Developing a routine can serve as one of the best natural sleep remedies. Do your best to go to bed and wake up at the same time each day, since this works well with your internal body clock and helps to improve sleep.*

- *Avoid eating your dinner in a loud and noisy environment, as this can stimulate your mind and make it more difficult to sleep.*

- *Be mindful of what you are eating, and chew your food thoroughly. Chewing the food well before it enters the gut ensures proper digestion and good sleep.*

PHYSICAL EXERCISE

Physical exercise is one of the best natural sleep remedies, improving both the quality and quantity of sleep. Consider the following:

- *If your day job involves working at a desk, you will definitely need to incorporate a daily physical workout to ensure proper sleep.*
- *Engage in physical exercise in the morning, midday, or late afternoon, but avoid exercising late at night because exercise itself is a stimulant. It could potentially keep you wide awake if it's too close to your bedtime.*

MENTAL AND EMOTIONAL REST

The more you can give your mind and emotions a break, the better you will be able to sleep. The following recommendations can help quiet your mind:

- *One hour before bedtime, free yourself from office-related work, leave your phone and other gadgets aside, and allow your body and mind to slowly relax.*
- *Light activates your brain, so darken your bedroom an hour before bedtime. Even a small streak of light can destroy the sleep-inducing neurochemical melatonin, resulting in sleep disturbances.*
- *Briefly recall all the incidents, encounters, and any emotional turmoil from your day. Now let them go and experience lightness in mind and body.*

- *Ayurveda and Yoga recommend activities such as meditation, light reading, or a mindfulness technique to induce sleep.*

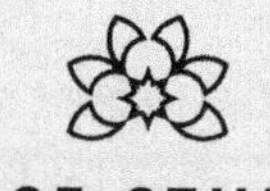

CASE STUDY

Diana, a mother of two young children, visited my office for assistance. Ever since her children were born, she lived in a constant state of sleep deprivation. At first, it was the normal new-mom period of nighttime wakings, feeding the baby, etc. Even several years later, she found that she never returned to a normal sleeping pattern. Diana found herself becoming forgetful, irritable, and clumsy. Knowing that years of sleep deprivation were closely linked to the negative mental and physical effects she was experiencing, she asked for advice to end the cycle of poor sleep, mood swings, stress, more bad sleep, etc.

Diana began to follow some of my dietary recommendations, cutting out caffeine after 10 a.m. and giving herself several hours after eating dinner before retiring to bed. She made an effort to reduce her intake of greasy, sugary, and processed foods—and did the same when she prepared food for the family. She also began to incorporate long walks with her dog into the daily routine.

A few hours before bedtime, she would turn off her phone, dim the lights, and read to her children – followed by some light reading herself. As she prepared for bed, she spent a few minutes breathing gently as she engaged in a brief meditation. She envisioned any stressful events from the day and allowed her mind to gently release them.

Within a few weeks, Diana began sleeping more soundly, waking up in the middle of the night less and less, until she finally began sleeping through the entire night. And within a few months, her typical six-hours-a-night of sleep increased to seven or eight. As these changes to her sleep occurred, she noticed immediate mental benefits as well. Diana felt refreshed in the morning and much more optimistic. Her brain-fog lifted, and she had more patience with her husband and children. As for the clumsiness? Diana felt more levelheaded and clear-minded and ceased tripping and dropping things.

Additional Tips from the GLP Toolbox on Sleep

Follow these additional tips for even more ideas that will improve your sleep each night:

- *Drink a soothing cup of warm, organic cow's milk or almond milk before bed. Add a pinch of ground nutmeg to calm the nervous system. As an alternative to milk, sip some chamomile, valerian, or spearmint tea.*

- *Listen to soft music in the evening as part of your bedtime routine.*

- *Gently massage your temples, eyes, and the soles of your feet with coconut or sesame oil that contains a few drops of cedar-wood, valerian, or lavender essential oil.*

- *To meditate, sit perfectly still for a few minutes. Take several slow, deep breaths as you watch your thoughts flow by naturally. Don't focus on any single thought, but instead notice the thoughts and then gently release them. This practice can steadily relax the body and prepare it for sleep.*

- *Ensure a bedroom temperature between sixty-five- and seventy-degrees Fahrenheit (eighteen and twenty-two degrees Celsius) to drift off to sleep faster.*

Reminder: For optimal results, continue to integrate the practices from all previous and future chapters into your daily routine. The more practices you can include in your life, the more results you will see!

CHAPTER 6

SELFLESS SERVICE

"Therefore without any attachment, without interruption, perfectly perform selfless actions by which a person attains the highest good."

THE BHAGAVAD GITA, CHAPTER 3, VS. 19.

One of the ways to achieve well-being at the level of body and mind, while also cultivating contentment and sustaining mental health, is through the path of selfless service. When a person provides selfless service —*seva* in Sanskrit, *karma yoga* in the Yoga philosophy—he or she does so without any egoistic tendencies, whether it is providing finances to support an orphanage or a food bank, helping a someone who's blind to cross the road, mentoring a student without seeking fees, etc.

To render selfless service, you must develop two qualities: overcoming attachment to the specific task and cultivating a loving attitude to perform the selfless service. In other words, you must have no expectations after rendering the selfless service, and you must remain unaffected by the results while maintaining a loving attitude. If you do not love to render selfless service and do so only out of a sense of compulsion, this creates a conflict in your mind, which can lead to emotional upheaval.

As you begin to decide how you can perform a selfless service, learn to create love towards the duty first. Let go of the ego, including feelings of desire, ambition, fear, worry, anxiety, judgment, and anger to release any attachments to the service or its outcome.

You will know when you are rendering selfless service because you will experience a state of high prana. You'll feel peaceful, calm, nonjudgmental, and neutral. By focusing on the selfless action alone, you will enter this high-prana state and encourage your physical, mental, and emotional growth.

Scientifically speaking, selfless service also has additional benefits. Numerous scientific articles on selfless service conclude that a strong correlation exists between the well being, happiness, health, and longevity of people who render selfless service without any expectation, as long as they feel good about performing these tasks. Researchers report that adults who perform selfless service experience less depression, greater life satisfaction, and more happiness, thereby leading to improvements in overall health.[118]

Below are some additional benefits derived from selfless service:

WARDS OFF DEPRESSION

Selfless service protects the doer from depression. In any selfless service setting, social interaction and cooperation are integral components of the service. Engaging in a social network with others toward a common cause helps reduce isolation and thereby overcome depression.[119]

BUILDS SELF-ESTEEM

Performing a selfless service without any expectation helps to build esteem and self-confidence.[120]

INCREASES LIFESPAN

Those of us who perform selfless service regularly live longer compared to those who do not. In one longitudinal study involving high school graduates from 1957, researchers caught up with over 3,000 of these people at ages sixty-five and older. They found that those who had performed selfless service regularly lived longer compared with those who did not. Additionally, the participants who rendered the service only for compassionate reasons achieved the most health benefits compared to those who performed the service purely for personal gain or self-growth.[121] According to one of the authors of this study, "*Our research implies that should any benefits to the self become the main motive for performing selfless service, the doer may not see the health benefits associated with the selfless service.*"

In another study, researchers found that selfless service in the form of giving time and assistance reduced mortality rates, independent of other confounding factors, including health practices and social support. Subjects who volunteered for two or more causes had a 63 percent lower rate of mortality compared to non-volunteers.[122]

RELEASES POSITIVE HORMONES

While performing a selfless service, the body releases several important hormones, including dopamine, oxytocin, and endorphins. These "feel-good" hormones assist in buffering stressful thoughts, allowing the person to enter a state of euphoria, tranquility, serenity, and inner peace. Actually, just thinking about a selfless service can releases these "feel-good" chemicals, too.[123] If you're familiar with the term "runner's high" (the state of euphoria, feelings of being invincible, reduced state of discomfort and pain, loss in the sense of time, etc.), that is how you will feel when performing a selfless act. Some even describe reductions in anxiety levels and more positive feelings towards the self and the world. In other words, it's a win-win for both the doer and receiver.[124]

The benefits of selfless service do not come by simply offering a few pennies to charity. True selfless service and its benefits result from going that extra mile: sacrificing time and effort.[125] In several studies, benefits from selfless service were seen only among those participants who volunteered at least an hour of work once a month, or those who offered their services more frequently.[126] The health benefits from selfless service are so profound that the United Nations and several European governments are encouraging citizens to volunteer and render selfless service.

Some of my students complain that they have stopped offering their charitable services because the receiver did not put it to good use. Some have noticed that the money they offered to the homeless was used for smoking or to buy drugs. In these cases, the doer has forgotten a tenet of selfless service—to carry out the act, and that's it. There cannot be any expectation after rendering the service, and doers are neither responsible nor answerable to the receiver's actions following the selfless act.

Some Personal Stories of Selfless Service

My father instilled in me the virtue of performing voluntary duties as he believed in giving without any thought of recognition or gain. He believed in the virtue of giving rather than receiving. Thanks to his noble deeds and influence, I began performing selfless acts as a teenager. After my classes ended, I would stay after school and help the teachers or tutor several primary school students. For several students who were blind, I would read the chapters of textbooks to them, or scribe for them as they dictated answers to exams. Over the weekend, I assisted at our city library by sorting and cataloging books. As I got older, I organized numerous camps to provide food and clothing to the homeless and destitute.

Next, I began to extend selfless service in those areas where humans feared to tread. For instance, on the outskirts of the city where I lived, there was a community of people afflicted with leprosy. Leprosy is a chronic bacterial disease that primarily affects the skin, peripheral nerves, mucosa of the upper respiratory tract, and the eyes. The disease is contagious and transmitted via droplets from the nose and mouth. People afflicted with this disease are ostracized by the family and shunned by the community, so they will seek shelter within their fraternity, living in far-flung areas of the city with minimal contact with mainstream people. I organized monthly social and relief work at these leprosy camps by distributing food, arranging for medical aid, and teaching health and hygiene-awareness programs.

Since that time, it's been a long journey of numerous selfless acts. I do so primarily because I place the well-being of others as a top priority ahead of personal gain or achievement, and because I love performing these selfless duties. Selfless service is a decision that I chose, and coupling it with loving-kindness and empathy makes a huge impact in my life. Life is a journey of opposites, and, like everyone else in the world, I too experience difficult choices, stressful events, and challenging situations. But simple acts of selfless service continue to make me stronger and give me a deeper sense of self-confidence that I can make it through turbulent phases seamlessly. Selfless acts have helped me to follow the path of love and selflessness, and this is a path that I enjoy to live.

I share these details not to show off or brag, but rather to give you ideas that may spark your own path of selfless service. I hope that in sharing these experiences, you are convinced that the benefits of providing these services are real and will benefit both you and the receiver, making the world a better place.

Going One Step Further: Altruistic Behavior

There is another aspect of selfless service: altruistic behavior. Altruistic behavior involves rendering selfless acts in extraordinary ways by sacrificing time, energy, resources, and often *your own life*—even though you may not receive anything in return. How do we explain this altruistic behavior when someone puts others' welfare ahead of his or her own?

Evolutionary biologists are intrigued by the fact that natural selection favors this type of behavior, and these actions are displayed among humans and animals alike. One possible explanation is that an exemplary selfless act benefits the kin or society at large, even if it is at the expense of the altruist's own life.[127] Imagine a setting where several people render selfless acts—even if they are required to sacrifice their own lives. In these instances, more people benefit from this cooperation, and these positive effects would extend to society through generations, thereby paving the way for a better world in which to live.[128]

The notable yoga teacher, Mr. B.K.S. Iyengar, alludes to selfless service and altruistic behavior when he couples the benefits of compassion to selfless service that relieves misery or suffering. He believes that a true altruist is one who, without any expectation or reward, uses all the available resources to mitigate pain, misery, and suffering, and provides courage and strength to the weak, as well as shelter to all. In doing so, the doer of the service overcomes emotional, mental, and physical turbulence. Ultimately, the act becomes intrinsically rewarding.[129]

Selfless service is one of the core values of the defense forces of every country. A soldier who gives his or her life to protect the country is exhibiting an altruistic behavior, even if he or she is no longer present to receive recognition or acknowledgment. And yet, we live in a society where the anticipated reward that motivates most charitable giving is the fame, credit, and acclaim that follows the act. However, by shifting your priorities toward a mindset of selfless service, you can escape the world's fleeting moments of "success" and know that you are making a difference that will extend far into the future.

Tips from the GLP Toolbox on Selfless Service

When contemplating how you can perform selfless service, consider the following information and tips:

- *Do not resort to selfless service as a stand-alone tool for good health and wellness. This must be combined with good eating practices, physical exercise, tuning the senses, maintaining a good sleeping practice, and keeping your mind sharp. Review the recommendations in Chapters 1-5 for more information.*

- *An easy way to get started is to mentor a neighbor or relative's son or daughter. If there are expenses that a child cannot afford (education, extra-curricular activities, etc.), consider helping that child (and his or her family) with the cost.*

- *Teach a language for free to people who cannot speak the language fluently.*

- *Provide any kind of free service to prison inmates.*

- *On your birthday, give something to the needy instead of waiting to receive something.*

- *Pick up random trash as you walk down the street or in a park.*

- *Help the needy cross busy intersections.*

- *Commemorate the death anniversary of a loved one by providing a warm, fresh meal to the homeless or others in need. This not only helps the receivers but also adds meaning to your loved one's death.*

- *The next time you hear a fire truck or ambulance siren—or see these emergency service vehicles on the road—silently wish that these vehicles reach their destination safely. Give a blessing for the firefighters/paramedics to provide aid on time to the distressed folks. Pray that the injured individuals do not experience too much pain or suffering and receive help ASAP.*

- *If you perform a selfless service, silently wish that any benefit from your charitable act goes to another individual who needs it the most.*

- *Help any person with disabilities or special needs.*
- *Donate your hair to organizations that can turn your locks into wigs for cancer patients.*
- *Educate the illiterate for free.*
- *Make regular, anonymous charitable donations.*
- *Donate cash or clothes without claiming a tax exemption.*
- *Walk shelter dogs at the humane society.*

Reminder: For optimal results, continue to integrate the practices from all previous and future chapters into your daily routine. The more practices you can include in your life, the more results you will see!

PART III

GOOD EMOTIONAL PRACTICES

The mind and emotions are distinct yet related entities. Good Emotional Practices involve using effective tools to perceive, understand, control, evaluate, and express your emotions so that you become more conscious of life's challenges, while at the same time increasing your capacity for controlling emotional upheavals. This enhanced awareness and understanding of your emotions enable you to experience complete peace and joy as your creativity unfolds.

GOOD EMOTIONAL PRACTICES INCLUDE THE FOLLOWING:

CHAPTER 7: MEDITATION

During meditation, your mind remains undistracted and still for a length of time, and your emotional state is calm and balanced in those moments as well. Meditation is a combination of undivided attention, focus, and awareness. The end result is a complete integration of the body, mind, and emotions. Meditation can also bring about feelings of fulfillment and achievement.

CHAPTER 8: CULTIVATING THE NOBLE FIVE

We carry with us an enormous amount of emotional baggage, which weighs us down, clouding our emotions, perception, and awareness. Over time, failure to release those negative feelings can lead to mental illnesses and chronic physical conditions. Cultivating the noble five—a defined set of positive emotions—helps to welcome desirable thoughts that fetch unlimited happiness, satisfaction, clarity, and joy.

CHAPTER 9: OVERCOMING THE DETERRENTS

Emotional obstacles may prevent you from leading a peaceful life, and this may result in repeated pain, suffering, dissatisfaction, and delusion. Overcoming these deterrents is the key to living a more peaceful, fulfilled life at all three levels: body, mind, and emotions.

CHAPTER 7

MEDITATION

"The continuous flow of the same thought or image of the object of focus, without being distracted by any other thought is meditation."

YOGA SUTRAS ON EXPERIENCES
VIBHUTI PAADA, CHAPTER 3

Each one of us is made up of a physical body, a mental body, and an emotional body. However, if we live with the idea that these entities are completely independent of one another, we will experience suffering and ill health. Instead of compartmentalizing the three, it is important to understand that they are integrated.

Good Emotional Practices are all about cultivating harmonious thoughts and discarding negativity to reduce mental conflict and promote a fully functional, healthy life. Your thoughts are extremely powerful as they control your psyche and have the ability to nurture or destroy you. A thought is like a seed, so if you nourish and water it daily with positivity, it will grow and branch out constructively. It is for this reason that positive thoughts keep you happy and content, while disharmonious thoughts place you in a downward spiral of poor health and suffering.

In addition to your own happiness and contentment, thoughts can also influence others. For this reason, be mindful of the thoughts you hold for others. Negative thoughts directed at other people can have a deleterious impact on both you and the other person. It works the same when sending out harmonious thoughts to others, which will nurture positive feelings in them and yourself.

One simple tool that allows us to absorb harmonious thoughts and flush out negative ones is meditation. Meditation lets you clear your mind, release emotional drama, and improve your focus without resistance. In his book, *Flow*, Mihaly Csikszentmihalyi alludes to the benefits of meditation and Good Emotional Practices in his definition of being in a state of flow: "*When an individual is engaged in an activity that has clear goals and which requires specific responses, that is, when a person's skills are fully involved in overcoming a challenging task, the individual has an undivided focus and gets totally involved and forgets everything else but the activity.*"[130]

A good example of the concept of flow is the undisturbed concentration you may exhibit while preparing for an exam. Nothing perturbs you because you're fully focused, and your mind is completely absorbed in the coursework. In this example, you have entered a kind of meditative state with your studies. Military personnel can experience flow as well. For instance, snipers describe their feelings of focus as they channel their attention and awareness on the target for a sustained period. This is a form of meditation. Even something as simple as intently watching a glass of milk in the microwave oven so it doesn't boil over is a form of focused, meditative action.

A meditative state is not restricted to any particular activity, and it occurs in different ways for different people. In addition to the aforementioned examples, you may experience a meditative state while playing a sport, playing music, reading, painting, drawing, or writing. Simply put, when your emotional state is calm, free from drama, and still, you are meditating. While it may sound like an effortless state, meditation actually requires discipline and effort to access it. However, its benefits are worth the effort, as you will learn in the next section.

The Benefits of Meditation

Advances in neuroimaging have enabled scientists to study and identify the dramatic quieting of several areas of the brain in those who meditate. Using state-of-the-art imaging techniques, researchers are confirming meditation's positive effects on the brain's structure, behavior, and function. Meditation appears to have an amazing variety of benefits:[131]

- *Reduces fear, worry, anxiety, anger, and rage*
- *Reduces chronic pain*
- *Increases cognitive function*

- *Lowers blood pressure*
- *Alleviates post-traumatic stress syndrome*
- *Slows down cellular aging*
- *Reduces pain perception, through a dampening of the brain's pain receptors*
- *Reduces inflammation*

For those suffering from age-associated memory impairment, meditation reverses hippocampal (an area of the brain involved with memory) degeneration. At the same time, meditation can improve neuronal branching and connectivity, suggesting meditation's role in neuroplasticity.[132] As previously discussed in Part II, the brain is constantly changing, modulating, and rewiring itself in response to new experiences, leading to stronger and more permanent neuronal branches.

In addition to neuroplasticity and branching, research studies show that participants with more than twenty years of meditation experience have more gray matter volume throughout the brain. The gray matter contains mostly neuronal and non-neuronal cells, and it is chiefly related to muscle control and sensory perception – including seeing and hearing, memory, emotions, speech, decision-making, and self-control. The volume of the gray matter is a measure of the density of brain cells, and it appears to correlate positively with various abilities and skills. As we age, we experience significant loss in our gray matter volume, which means we lose some of the functions associated with those specific areas of the brain.[133]

Age-associated gray matter decline is significant in the memory centers of the brain (the hippocampus and entorhinal cortex), which can lead to dementia. However, long-term meditators—when compared to non-meditators—had more well-preserved brains, with smaller reductions in brain volume.[134] The aging process also affects normal cerebral blood flow, and this, in turn, triggers gray matter loss and dysfunction. But when it comes to meditation, several studies report that this practice triggers increased cerebral blood flow, leading to improved moods for the participants.[135] Understanding how meditation affects the entire brain, then, may partially explain the brain's resilience exhibited by seasoned meditators.

Am I Meditating... Or Not?

People commonly ask how to differentiate between a meditative and non-meditative state. While the experience can be subjective, a meditative state can be confirmed by observing brainwave patterns. Brainwaves are electrochemical signals generated by neurons that are the basis for motor functions, thoughts, emotions, and behavior, and their patterns can be detected by placing sensors on the head. These waves are bandwidths that change according to our behavior and emotions. Slower brainwave patterns indicate that someone is tired, fatigued, sluggish, slow, or dreamy. Meanwhile, fast brainwave patterns correlate to alert, fast-paced, and hyper-moody behavior.

Brainwaves can be broken down further into the following types:

DELTA WAVES

These low-frequency, high-amplitude, deeply penetrating, and slow brainwaves are generated during deep meditation and dreamless sleep. The presence of delta waves indicates that the individual is unaffected by external impressions.

THETA WAVES

Theta brainwaves appear most often in dream sleep, as well as together with delta waves during deep meditation. Mental and emotional tasks such as learning, memory acquisition, intuition, and nightmares are characterized by the presence of theta waves.

ALPHA WAVES

Living in the present (also known as being in the "here and now") marks the appearance of alpha brainwaves. They would appear after you have just completed a task, sit down to rest, take time out to reflect, or take a break to walk in silence.

BETA WAVES

Beta brainwaves are fast-acting and dominate during the waking state. They are also operational when you are alert, attentive, and engaged in mental activity.

Researchers have shown that even though one specific brainwave may dominate during any given activity, the remaining brainwaves will continue to be present—albeit at low levels. While all four brainwaves work in tandem, studies show that meditation is associated with increased delta and theta brainwave patterns. This supports the use of meditation as an intervention tool for those with emotional, mental, and physical health issues, including depression, anxiety, mood disorders, sensory pain, and physical impairment.

Feelings During Meditation

According to Yoga philosophy, several aspects of one's individuality emerge during meditation, including greater awareness, improved attention, and sustained concentration. Therefore, as you let the flood of emotions go, you will become more aware and attentive, for a sustained period. As you prepare to meditate, offer the intention of developing strong, undistracted focus. This will silence your mind chatter, leading to a more peaceful yet fully aware mind.

Note the feelings you will begin to experience when you're in a truly meditative state:

- *Losing feelings of self-consciousness*
- *Losing your sense of time*
- *Becoming unaware of physical needs and mental cravings*
- *Experiencing intrinsically-rewarding feelings*
- *Feeling a state of clarity and control over a situation and its outcome*
- *Experiencing a neutral emotional state and disposition*

Knowing how important meditation is to your brain and emotional state, let's get started with some easy ways to incorporate meditation with the other Good Living Practices from Parts I and II.

Meditation and Other Good Living Practices

When it comes to Good Physical Practices and meditation, let's start with your diet. By eating a high prana food, you can become aware of what, why, how, where, and when you are eating that food. Also, one of the Good Living Practices requires you to maintain undivided attention, focus, and awareness on your food, transforming your eating into a meditative act.

Physical exercise of any kind is the perfect meditative activity. If you focus your attention and awareness on the exercise, you are engaging in the act of meditation. The combination of focus, breath work, precise alignment, and the controlling power of how hard you're pushing yourself not only allow you to match the challenge to your skill level but also put you in a state of meditative flow. These experiences will lead to feelings of accomplishment and happiness while simultaneously improving your health.

Regular self-care and tuning of the sense organs is another meditative act, as it requires you to become fully aware of how your senses are functioning. Through your focused attention and awareness, you will experience feelings of harmony and happiness. And the more harmonious your life becomes, the healthier your body, mind, and emotional state will become, with minimal discomfort and suffering.

In Part II, you learned about the importance of keeping your mind and brain strong and resilient. By learning new things, engaging in different hobbies and interests, and challenging yourself through mentally stimulating activities, you will keep the brain growing strong. At the same time, these mental exercises require awareness, attention, and sustained focus, which places you in a meditative state.

Quality sleep and meditation go hand in hand because both require the individual to remain still, calm, and peaceful. I'm sure you've experienced sleepless nights when you're feeling agitated or if there is a lot of drama in your life. Meditating for a few moments before bed can help you to release those negative emotions while improving sleep quality. An added bonus is that your undisturbed sleep will also become a form of meditation, too.

Selfless service is also a meditative act because for the service to succeed, it requires a single focus, feeling of peacefulness, and a commitment to remain unaffected by the results.

Clearly, the Good Physical Practices and Good Mental Practices described here need to be performed as meditative exercises to reap the maximum benefits. But what happens when you're not engaged in any of those tasks? How does meditation work in these situations? The next section will describe different types of meditation, as well as each method's benefits.

Types of Meditation

While the classical Yoga or Vedic texts discuss just one kind of meditation (generally known as the yogic meditation), a variety of meditation techniques have evolved. Regardless of what type of meditation it is, the basic premise remains the same: letting go of the emotions, stilling the mind, relaxing the body, drawing focus inward, and sustained concentration.

While teachers, books, and other forms of literature may declare that their style of meditation is correct and dismiss other forms of meditation as incorrect or unsafe, my suggestion is to try out all the different types and see what resonates with you. Any claim that there is only one real way to meditate is incorrect. Remember, no single style is special or particularly better, or right or wrong. You must find the type that meets your needs and aligns with your nature.

I suggest you try one meditation method for a couple of weeks, and if it does not align with your inner instincts, switch to a different meditation technique. Regardless of the practice you choose, it is important to avoid resisting the disturbing and distracting influences that attempt to get in your way during meditation. If your mind wanders, be aware of what's happening and simply return to your point of focus— the breath. Do not try to resist or block out mental fluctuations that invade the mind because resistance will only create more resistance, resulting in frustration. Instead, simply let the invasive thoughts be as you continue with the meditation.

If you are a novice, I would suggest you meditate for two minutes each morning. If you can relax and sit still, move to four minutes. Keep increasing your time as you become more comfortable with the practice. If too many dramas play in your mind, simply acknowledge them and try to let go of all the internal chatter. Use your breath as a point of focus and keep coming back to it each time your mind strays away. Remember that everything is a part of meditation: the noise, thoughts, emotions, and mental resistance. Understanding this will allow you to relax, return to your breath, and enter an even deeper state of stillness!

Once you start your daily practice of meditation, sustain the practice, and keep it going. After a month of steady practice, notice what impact the practice of meditation had on your body, mind, and emotions. Meditation is like learning and becoming competent in a new skill. The more and longer you meditate, the more impact it will have on your health and wellbeing.[136] Check the GLP Toolkit at the end of this chapter for more tips on meditation.

While there are several resources available about the different types of meditation, I will just be listing a subset of them.

MINDFULNESS MEDITATION

This form of meditation encourages you to remain aware and be present in the moment. As you meditate mindfully, you encourage your thoughts to flow while your mind remains active. At the same time, you are keeping yourself in the present, neither dwelling on the past nor thinking about the future. In this meditative state, your body, mind, and emotions unite as one entity, and you will begin to feel intrinsically rewarded.

Evidence of mindfulness meditation can be witnessed through the compositions of musical maestros like Bach and Beethoven, the artwork of Da Vinci and Picasso, and the performances of opera singers. These individuals would have been operating in a meditative state of flow as they immersed themselves in their work. Fortunately, this type of meditation is not reserved for exceptional artists; anyone can meditate mindfully. In fact, many people are drawn to mindfulness meditation, and numerous evidence-based research studies encourage this type of practice.[137]

TRANSCENDENTAL MEDITATION

Transcendental meditation is a silent form of mantra meditation, a spiritual form introduced by Maharishi Mahesh Yogi. In this technique, you remain seated while focused on a mantra (a repeated word or series of words). As you meditate, you allow the sounds of the mantra to coincide with your breathing.[138]

BODY SCANNING

While mindfulness and transcendental meditation can be performed with the eyes open, a body scan—also known as progressive relaxation—is performed with your eyes closed and your body flat (or sitting in a comfortable, upright position). In this meditation, you start with your feet, scanning for any feelings of tension, which you then release. Afterward, you continue to move your awareness up and throughout your entire body. As you scan each part, notice any stiffness, achiness, or tension—and then overcome it by relaxing the muscles surrounding that area.[139]

PASSAGE MEDITATION

This form of meditation, developed by the famous spiritual guru, Eknath Eswaran, and first taught systematically at the University of California, Berkeley, involves fully immersing yourself into a scriptural passage without disturbance or distraction. The key is to repeat the passage verbally or mentally many times until it eventually transforms your character, conduct, and consciousness.[140]

YOGIC MEDITATION

Now, imagine trying to achieve a meditative state—except that you are only focusing on your inhalation and exhalation. Let go of all physical action and mental drama as you become aware of the sounds of your breath. While the stillness in your physical body sets in and the mental chatter in your mind dampens, gently notice if your focus and concentration are directed toward your breath. If you can sustain this state, you have achieved the yogic meditation state—also known as the Zen state. This is a feeling of stillness characterized by the union of the body, mind, and emotions, into a state of equanimity—a single entity, fully engaged in the sounds of the breath. The goal is to feel at ease, relaxed, and at peace with yourself and your surroundings.[141]

TWIN HEARTS MEDITATION

This is a powerful meditation technique practiced by Pranic healers. Pranic healing is a therapeutic, non-touch energy healing modality in which the practitioner uses energy or life force to balance the body, mind, and emotions, thereby improving health. Twin hearts meditation allows practitioners and healers to amplify the inner energy for their own healing as well as regulate and direct this energy to heal beings worldwide.[142]

Resources

Below is a list of various meditation resources. I have visited a few of these places, but other than that, I do not hold any specific affiliation with the centers listed below. I encourage you to check for other specific meditation centers in your area.

1. **Spirit Rock Meditation Center (**www.spiritrock.org**)**

    Set in the secluded hills of West Marin County, California, Spirit Rock Meditation Center offers a supportive environment and a variety of programs for the practices of insight, mindfulness, and loving-kindness meditation.

2. **Silent Stay Meditation & Retreat Center** (www.silentstay.com)

    This retreat center supports people of all denominations to live a meaningful life through the path of meditation encompassing devotion, simplicity, humility, and service to others.

3. **Transcendental Meditation Retreat** (www.miravalarizona.com)

    Tucked in the warm shade of Tucson's Santa Catalina Mountains, this retreat offers an array of mindful programs to increase physical, mental, and emotional health.

4. **Blue Mountain Center of Meditation** (www.bmcm.org):

    Nestled in the long, narrow inlet of the Pacific Ocean, this nonprofit organization founded by Eknath Easwaran offers publications, activities, and programs based on the eight-point program of passage meditation that Easwaran proposed.

5. **Shambhala Mountain Center** (www.shambhalamountain.org)

    Nestled high in the Colorado Rockies, Shambhala Mountain Center offers a supportive environment to meditate, connect with community and develop mindful-awareness and compassion.

6. **Anubhuti Meditation & Retreat Center** (www.anubhutiretreatcenter.org)

    The Anubhuti Retreat Center in Marin County, created by the Brahma Kumaris World Spiritual Organization, offers several programs on raja yoga meditation that helps individuals understand their inner strengths and values.

7. **Transcendental Meditation** (www.tm.org/enlightenment):

   Founded by Maharishi Mahesh Yogi, this form of meditation promotes a state of relaxed awareness by transcending thoughts and other mental dramas.

8. **Meditation Reading Resources – Ten Percent Happier** (www.tenpercent.com/reading):

   This is a one-stop resource for books and literature on meditation.

9. **50 Best Meditation Books (**www.positivepsychology.com/meditation-books/**):**

   This is a one-stop resource for books and literature on meditation.

Tips from the GLP Toolkit

Without undivided attention, focus, and awareness, you will not be effective at any task or project at home, school, or work. To be as efficient and effective as possible, you must work on cultivating a meditative state. Whether it's an exam, interview, surgical procedure, musical performance, artistic creation, etc., all tasks can be performed at a consistently high level when done so meditatively. Here are some tips to help you enhance, fine-tune, and maintain your meditative practices:

If you've never meditated before, start small. Personally, I begin my practice by engaging in meditation for five minutes, three times each day. Early-morning meditation helps my day begin on a positive note, while a quick meditation at noon helps maintain peace and calm. Meanwhile, the evening meditation allows me to settle down after a full day of events.

If you find yourself in slow-moving traffic, practice meditation by calmly noticing your surroundings. Study the different vehicles, colors, sizes, and shapes. Allow yourself to become absorbed within the moment. To do this safely, remain aware of the cars in the rear and ahead of you, as well as the distance between one another. As you drive, maintain focus on the road and vehicles surrounding you without distraction.

Whatever you do at home or outside, approach each activity in a meditative way. This will help you make meditation part of your lifestyle, leading to a union of the body, mind, and emotions.

Here are some final reminders about achieving that meditative state in tandem with practices that nurture your body, mind, and emotions:

Be aware of what, why, how, where, and when you eat. As you sit and eat, sustain undivided attention, focus, and awareness on your food.

Before eating, bless and thank the elements and beings that contributed to the plate of food in your presence. The Vedic texts provide one simple mantra to give thanks to all: "*Annadhata Sukhi Bhava.*" Thank the universe, rain, sun, the farmer, plants, animals, traders, and cook. This is a simple yet powerful meditative act.

Engage in any type of physical exercise with attention, focus, and awareness to achieve "meditation in action."

Be meditative while caring for your five senses by being fully aware of their functions and applying the practices in Chapter 3 to tune them in a healthy way.

- *Engage in mental exercises with awareness and focus to realize the greatest benefits.*

- *Improve your sleep practice, as meditation coupled with better sleep positively reinforces one another.*

- *Be sure that you remain detached from results during selfless service.*

- *As you become better at meditation in all aspects of your life, challenge yourself to practice yogic meditation—undivided attention, focus, and awareness on the breath alone.*

- *Once you become successful at yogic meditation, take it to the next level by practicing in an environment with loud noises, uncomfortable temperatures, strong aromas, etc.*

- *The next time you hear a fire truck or ambulance siren—or see these emergency service vehicles on the road—close your eyes briefly and direct your energy towards the emergency vehicle and its occupants. Silently wish that these vehicles reach their destination safely.*

  Send a blessing to the firefighters/paramedics to provide aid on time to the distressed folks. Direct your meditative energy towards the injured individuals and silently wish that they receive help ASAP.

- *As you continue onto Chapters 8 and 9, you will learn how meditation also keeps you in a positive state and increases your ability to overcome negative emotions.*

Reminder: For optimal results, continue to integrate the practices from all previous and future chapters into your daily routine. The more practices you can include in your life, the more results you will see!

CHAPTER 8

CULTIVATING THE NOBLE FIVE

"The greatest discovery of all time is that a person can change his future by merely changing his attitude."

OPRAH WINFREY

Good Emotional Practices include the cultivation of harmonious thoughts and feelings to reduce mental conflict while promoting a disease-free, fully functional, healthy life. Emotions can be a state, feeling, attitude, or response to an action, situation, or object. Emotions—especially negative ones—play a significant role in our daily lives, allowing us to be aware of and attentive to the triggers that create them.

Emotions can be seeded, nourished, and allowed to flourish. Just as a well-nurtured seed produces healthy leaves, stems, flowers, and fruits, feelings that we nurture turn into full-fledged emotions. Positive emotions should be encouraged and fostered since they shift the predominant beta brain waves that keep us aroused and alert into alpha waves that put us in the state of flow, which is characterized by a state of improved focus, concentration, and performance. This is also the state where our brains release feel-good chemicals like endorphins, noradrenaline, and dopamine. Positive emotions alter the energy patterns so that the mind, body, and emotions become unified and enter a high-prana state.

Other benefits of positive emotions include an overall reduction in stress, which promotes good health. That's because positive emotions soak up any stressful events and allow the individual to recover from the negative effects of stress more quickly. This, in turn, leads to an ability to manage and preserve mental and physical health more efficiently and effectively.[143] Positive emotions also promote immune resistance and encourage individuals to make sound, healthy decisions, which also lead to optimal health and wellness.

Check out the many benefits of positive emotions:

- *Happiness*
- *Contentment*

- *Effective coping skills*
- *Better psychological well-being, mental, and physical health*
- *A stronger, more resilient cardiovascular system*
- *Protection against memory loss*
- *Improvements in work life, social relationships, and job satisfaction*
- *Optimal lifespan*

Cultivating Positivity

Since it's important to remain in a positive emotional state, take time to consider the "noble five" emotional gems below. They can serve as an antidote to negative emotions and usher in unlimited happiness, love, compassion, and a state of oneness.[144]

CONTENTMENT

In the words of Patanjali, the Yoga philosopher, "*From an attitude of contentment, mental comfort, joy, and satisfaction are obtained.*" The word contentment has several synonyms, including happiness, satisfaction, fulfillment, pleasure, cheerfulness, gladness, gratification, ease, comfort, restfulness, well-being, peace, equanimity, serenity, and tranquility. Contentment is an emotional state where you feel happy with what you have—rather than looking at what's missing.

To be content, regardless of circumstance, can only be achieved when you can accept that there is a purpose for everything in your life. This allows you to process all experiences—both positive and negative—through a lens of satisfaction, knowing that everything in your life happens for a reason.

Sadly, too many people in today's world feel discontent, unhappy, and frustrated when they get caught up in a web of unfulfilled desires. Over time, this can lead to a loss of inner peace and disharmony in the physical body. However, if we can reverse these negative feelings and become content with what we currently have, the ego begins to fall away. This eventually leads to a state of oneness and unity, which contributes to a harmonious, healthy life.

If you don't currently feel content, is it worth the time and effort to work on this aspect of your emotional state? Absolutely! Contentment not only makes people happy and satisfied but also extends longevity, according to several research studies. One such study focused on subjective well-being (SWB) based on emotional factors like contentment, optimism, hopefulness, and sense of humor, among others. The conclusions were significant:[145]

- *People who are content exhibit a high SWB compared to those who are less content.*
- *Those with a high SWB had better overall health, and a high SWB closely correlated with a lower mortality rate.*
- *Unhappy and stressed people had low SWB levels, higher blood pressure levels, and lower immune responses, as compared to content people.*

An easy way to test your personal level of contentment is to determine if you are more influenced by material instincts and impulses, or if you regularly resist material temptations and instead find joy and satisfaction with your life—no matter where you are and what you're doing. If you find that you'd like to improve in this area, consider two elements of contentment: smiling and gratitude.

Imagine wearing a true smile, 24/7. This is universally evident among people who are content, and thus at peace. Smiles can be warm, beautiful, welcoming, cute, innocent, and/or melt your heart. Start smiling and people around you will brighten up and smile along with you. The world changes based on a person's perception and outlook, and having a smile will make you a pleasurable person to be around. A content person with a smile lights up the room, mitigates suffering, and elevates others' moods.

Those who sport a smile are considered more trustworthy, and people tend to help and cooperate with them more. Moreover, people who always smile are more stable (both mentally and physically), happier in their marriages, and they have better cognitive and interpersonal skills. Being content and smiling helps to boost the immune system, relieve stress, lower blood pressure, trigger the release of endogenous pain killers, and change one's attitude for the better.[146]

In addition to sporting a warm smile, people who are content also demonstrate appreciation. Being thankful and appreciative are virtues that define the act of gratitude. According to Yoga philosophy, contentment, smile, and gratitude always follow one another. An attitude of gratitude helps us to live life with a greater sense of well-being despite difficulties and disappointments. Cultivating this virtue benefits an individual because true gratitude releases the feel-good hormones which promote contentment and peace.[147]

True gratitude also increases and improves well being, health, the immune system, relationships, happiness levels, optimism, and empathy.[148] At the same time, gratitude counteracts any negativity, including dissatisfaction, displeasure, and unhappiness. In a research study conducted at UCLA, scientists used fMRI (functional magnetic resonance imaging) to measure the brain activity of subjects experiencing different emotions, and they found that gratitude activated several of the brain's reward regions simultaneously, similar to CNS drugs like Prozac.[149] However, unlike pharmaceuticals, the gratitude-associated brain changes lasted longer and did not trigger any nasty side effects.

According to Yoga philosophy, you must constantly seek opportunities to express your gratitude to experience good health and wellness. To that end, you may wish to practice gratitude as a form of meditation by affirming, "*I am content with life; I am smiling, life is good and rewarding, and I feel great about being here and now.*" You can also repeat the following: "*Let all beings experience peace, and only peace*" to express gratitude toward your loved ones, friends, colleagues, animals, birds, plants, and mother nature. In addition to your personal benefit, gratitude benefits the receiver. By "paying it forward," the recipient of your gratitude will pass the goodness along, creating a positive cycle of thanks.

FORGIVENESS

Louise Hay states, "*Forgiveness is for yourself because it frees you. It lets you out of that prison you put yourself in.*" No matter the mind-body therapy (Yoga, Ayurveda, pranic healing, etc.), they all impart a common, underlying principle: forgiveness. Forgiveness involves replacing painful memories with positive feelings and experiences. Forgiveness transforms negatives experiences, lessens the impact of traumatic events, and shifts the individual to a state of peace.

The fifth of the Ten Commandments of Yoga is *kshama*, which can be translated as forgiveness, forbearance, patience, or pardon. When we forgive, we can overcome sorrow, sadness, and negative memories. Forgiveness benefits the brain, too. Just as mentally stimulating exercise and meditation stimulate neuronal branching and new connections, forgiveness can improve connections, by trimming the neuronal branches associated with trauma. This ultimately prevents the reemergence of negative emotions from past experiences.[150]

A major challenge to the realization of inner peace is the inability to let go of hatred and bitterness. Forgiving someone who injured us—whether it was physical, mental, or emotional—can allow us to release painful, negative emotions. By forgiving, we are not excusing wrongdoing, letting the perpetrator "off the hook," or correcting the injustice; we are only freeing ourselves from the emotional bondage of the experience and moving forward, free and clear from those past events. It can be argued that forgiveness is a free gift to those who hurt us, yet the personal benefits that come from forgiving far outweigh any societal belief that we need to carry around resentment forever.

Although it may require effort, forgiveness comes more easily if you meditate on it. First, focus on forgiving and forgetting, and later commit all your energy to the process. With time, a favorable transformation will begin.

According to recent research studies, if you forgive and let go, you are likely to enjoy optimal blood pressure, a stronger immune system, and a drop in the stress hormones circulating in your blood. Other physical symptoms, like unexplained body pains, digestive issues, heart issues, and migraine headaches, could also subside.[151]

There is another important added benefit: living longer. In a study investigating the relationship between forgiveness and lifespan in a sample of 1,500 American adults aged sixty-six and older, researchers tested the benefits of forgiveness to longevity. The study followed the participants for three years to allow the researchers to determine whether forgiveness influenced health and mortality. After controlling for variables such as religion, social class, and health-related behaviors, the single parameter that greatly predicted mortality was the act of forgiveness. People who were averse to forgiving died earlier compared to people who were keen on forgiveness. The people who refused to forgive continued to harbor resentment and grudges, which eventually affected their overall health.[152]

On an emotional level, forgiving and letting go helps to curb negative emotions, including rage, anger, bitterness, resentment, and depression. It also allows the individual to recall positive aspects of an experience, despite any painful parts that existed simultaneously. According to one of the researchers on a forgiveness research project, "*Harboring unforgiveness comes at an emotional and a physiological cost. Cultivating forgiveness may cut these costs.*"[153]

HONESTY

"*Honesty is more than not lying. It is truth telling, truth speaking, truth living, and truth loving,*" remarked James Faust, the famous American religious leader and lawyer. Honest people are often perceived as sincere, decent, upright, and righteous individuals who live lives of integrity. Honesty can serve as an antidote to lower base desires, such as hypocrisy, covetousness, greed, sensual desires, and an unhealthy attachment to the superficial.

Being honest comes from knowing yourself and honoring what you know to be true in any given moment. By cultivating honesty, inner truth will find its way from your heart into the hearts of others. Honesty is not only a moral trait but also a personal virtue.

Practicing honesty has several health benefits as well. Dr. Anita Kelly, a psychology professor at the University of Notre Dame, focuses on honesty, truth, and its impact on physical and mental health. In a study where she spent ten weeks tracking the health of hundreds of adults, she noticed that the health of the participants went down considerably when they told more lies. Study participants who told fewer and minor lies had few health complaints compared to ones in the lie group, who complained of being tense, melancholic, or suffering from sore throats and headaches. Not surprisingly, both mental and physical health improved when the participants in the lie group started being more honest and stopped lying.[154]

While little research has been conducted on the effects of lying on health and wellness, the conclusion from studies that do exist show that lying releases stress hormones that can harm physical, mental, and emotional health.[155] According to these studies, lying and its negative effects are a two-sided problem: liars create physical, mental, and emotional problems for themselves, and people with these underlying problems are also more likely to continue lying.[156]

Lies not only imprison an individual, but the more lies someone tells, the more difficult it becomes to cover these lies or prevent being discovered. As a result, all the physical, mental, and emotional energies are diverted into protecting those lies, keeping the person telling the lies in a state of constant fear and stress.

To live harmoniously, you must practice honesty on all levels—through your thoughts, actions, and words. This not only creates integrity and harmony for yourself, but it also provides a platform for honest and open communication with others. By practicing honesty daily, you will enjoy enhanced mental and physical well being, as well as the sense that you are leading a more fulfilling, meaningful life.

LOVING-KINDNESS

A tenet of Yoga philosophy is this: "*Focusing with perfect discipline, the mind becomes purified by cultivating feelings of loving-kindness.*" Known as *Maitri-karuna* in Sanskrit, *Checed* in Hebrew, and *Metta* in Buddhism, loving-kindness encompass feelings of affection, warm-heartedness, as well as being considerate, humane, and sympathetic toward others.

Loving-kindness allows us to appreciate what we have and what we can give. Living life with a spirit of loving-kindness also increases feelings of gratitude, and forgiveness comes more easily and without hesitation. Not only that, random acts of loving-kindness make a huge impact on others' lives, giving them a feeling of hope and confidence.

Like other Good Living Practices, loving-kindness can also be experienced as a meditative act since it requires undivided attention, focus, and awareness. First, the process involves drawing attention to the mind and heart while connecting to your own sense of peace, friendliness, and compassion. While you focus, meditate on—and direct your loving-kindness toward other benefactors, such as parents, siblings, friends, teachers, pets, or anyone who needs support. You may also wish to direct this energy toward someone you consider to be problematic or challenging. While it's not always easy, make attempts to direct loving-kindness to those who evoke anger, rage, fear, resentment, antagonism, or any other difficult emotion. As you direct loving-kindness to others, intend for the positive energy to be sustained, giving the receiver everlasting peace, good health, and wellness.

Note: While practicing loving-kindness on difficult individuals, if negative emotions surface, honor and appreciate your limits and redirect the meditation toward yourself. Then, try to redirect the energy back to the challenging person and notice any emotional shifts. Continue alternating the energy between yourself and this individual until you overcome any mental turbulence. With practice, you can actually reach a point where this individual no longer emotionally affects you.

There are many reasons to practice loving-kindness meditation.[157] For example, in one study, a loving-kindness meditation group that practiced regularly experienced less distress than non-practitioners. The regular-practice group also saw a significant decrease in inflammation and cellular stress response compared to the low-practice (or no-practice) groups.

However, the beneficial changes were seen only in those who actively engaged in this practice.

Using fMRI measurements, researchers also noticed that loving-kindness meditations impacted several important brain regions that are primarily involved with empathy and the ability to adjust to the emotional states of others.[158] Sometimes, we tend to think about ourselves more than others, but if we spend more time thinking about those around us, the world would be a better place. Loving-kindness will connect you to others in a unique way, and the more you engage in loving-kindness meditation, you'll find that you won't want to stop this powerful practice.

NONVIOLENCE

Another tenet of Yoga philosophy is that "*for an individual who becomes firmly grounded in nonviolence, other people who come near will naturally lose any feelings of hostility.*" Unfortunately, we live in a world where violence prevails. Recent studies have shown that the United States suffers from far more violent deaths than any other wealthy nation, with approximately six violent deaths per 100,000 residents and more violent deaths in men (homicide and suicide) compared to other countries.[159]

When we consider the following definition of violence, those numbers would certainly climb even higher; according to a report from the World Health Organization, violence is "*the intentional use of force or power on self or against a person or a group.*"[160] This could be physical, mental, or emotional violence, resulting in physical harm, injury or death, trauma, depression, or PTSD, and it can affect both the perpetrator and the victim. If we closely reflect on this definition, then the person who is extremely critical, judgmental, and negative towards himself, herself, or others, would be considered violent—just like a person who walks with a gun and randomly shoots people. Of course, these are extreme examples to varying degrees, yet both have committed forms of violence. While the negative person's mental violence leads to an emotional burden directed toward self or others, the criminal perpetrator's violence leads to mayhem and loss of life.

Sadly, violence of any kind has profound effects on the health of an individual. Studies have shown the following:[161]

- *The stress of being in an abusive relationship has an obvious physical and psychological impact, as it often increases one's vulnerability to illness and may cause the victim to be more susceptible to disease.*

- *Battered victims experience depression, feelings of low self-esteem, and helplessness, coupled with somatic complaints.*

- *Chronic abuse causes serious psychological harm, including panic disorders, phobias, anxieties, and depression that may last for years. A victim's ability to trust and form emotional attachments are also severely impacted.*

- *Victims often complain of enduring the effects of violence over many years, and some even develop extreme symptoms years later in response to earlier incidents.*

- *Violence severely impacts healthy aging.*

- *Children who are exposed to various violent childhood events suffer from all kinds of stressors that negatively affect their overall development. A longitudinal research study found that six or more particular types of adverse experiences during childhood reduce life expectancy by twenty years among adults.*[162]

The logical solution to this grave problem is shunning violence and cultivating an attitude of nonviolence. Most people experience a natural sense of inner peace when they are in contact with those who practice and preach nonviolence. In the presence of a nonviolent person, there is a natural tendency to give up hostilities, ill will, and aggression in return.

Nonviolence builds upon all of the aforementioned virtues and comes naturally to those that are honest, content, forgiving—and among those whose presence is filled with unbounded smiles, positivity, and loving-kindness. It is easier to nurture nonviolence when we accept events as they are, act with an open and loving heart, and replace violent tendencies with loving-kindness, gratitude, compassion, and truth. Practicing non-violence on oneself helps to cultivate similar feelings towards others. For these reasons, I believe that nonviolence provides physical and mental benefits and could be a key predictor in leading a happy, healthy life.[163]

Resources

Below is a list of resources on the concept of non-violence. As with the resources for meditation, I do not hold any specific affiliation with the centers listed below. I encourage you to check for other centers or resources.

1. **1. Season for Nonviolence – M.K. Gandhi Institute for Nonviolence (**www.gandhiinstitute.org/season-for-nonviolence/**):**

   The mission of this institute is to develop resources and skills for achieving a nonviolent, sustainable, and just world in support of people and their communities.

2. **Resource Center for Nonviolence** (rcnv.org/nonviolence)**:**

   This organization provides resources for practicing nonviolent social change and also supports the growth of nonviolent activists.

3. **The King Center** (www.thekingcenter.org/king-philosophy)**:**

   The King center uses the six principles of nonviolence and is committed to eradicating the triple evils of poverty, racism, and militarism.

4. **Metta Center for Nonviolence** (www.mettacenter.org/nonviolence/introduction)**:**

   The mission of this center is to invest in nonviolent alternatives. It offers training, webinars, or workshops on nonviolence ideals for community and skill-building.

5. **The Center for Nonviolent Communication** (www.cnvc.org)**:**

   Founded by Marshall Rosenberg, the Center for Nonviolent Communication offers international intensive training and certification in nonviolent communication and resources to make life wonderful for all.

6. **Richmond Peace Education Center** (www.rpec.org/about-us/peace-education-resources/nonviolent-philosophy-and-conflict-theory)**:**

   The RPEC offers youth programs, workshops, public events, and conflict resolution training in the areas of peaceful conflict resolution, social justice, and nonviolent social change.

7. **Nonviolence International** (www.nonviolenceinternational.net)**:**

   Through inspirational stories, Nonviolence International supports constructive, nonviolent campaigns all over the globe.

8. **Nonviolence in Community Life** (www.tamera.org/nonviolence)**:**

   The mission of this institute is to create "biotopes," an integrated and unified habitat where all life forms, including humans, animals, plants, sea life, and other beings co-exist peacefully and in harmony.

9. **PEACE Magazine** (www.peacemagazine.org)**:**

   This resource publishes articles on all aspects of nonviolence with emphasis on democracy, human rights, global warming, famine, pandemics, radiation exposure, cyberthreats, and disarmament.

10. **Books on Nonviolence** (www.goodreads.com/shelf/show/nonviolence):

    This is a one-stop resource for the most popular books on all forms of nonviolence.

11. **Resources about Nonviolence** (www.lutheran_peace.tripod.com/nonviolence)**:**

    A comprehensive resource center for all dimensions of nonviolence.

12. **Resources on nonviolence and just peace** (www.nonviolencejustpeace.net/resources)**:**

    This is one-stop resource center on nonviolence and just peace.

Tips from the GLP Toolbox for Noble Intentions

Cultivating the noble five and practicing these intentions daily is the basis for the physical and mental benefits that accompany these virtues. Be sure to combine these intentions with good eating, physical exercise, tuning of the five senses, and mental exercise for optimum results.

Follow these additional tips and reminders:

- *Cultivating the noble five can improve your sleep, improving conditions like sleep apnea, insomnia, and poor sleep quality.*[164]
- *Eating high-prana foods, drawing in harmonious impressions through your five senses, physical and mental exercise, meditation, and selfless service are some of the best tools to live a nonviolent life. Use these tools daily to reduce emotional drama and conflicts as well.*
- *Practicing the noble five with undivided attention, focus, and awareness will lead to success in any task or project.*
- *Remember that a calm, pure emotional state will inspire words and actions that resonate with your internal and external world.*
- *Be content with what you have or possess. If you have more than you need, donate the excess to charity.*
- *Always be grateful for something. Look for simple, small things in life that inspire happiness and give thanks.*
- *Avoid using negative language (like "life sucks") that dulls your sense of gratitude.*
- *Think of someone who has hurt you or whom you despise.*

Realize that holding onto resentment and hatred only invites disease and suffering into your life. Instead, be courageous and forgive that individual. This will free you to enjoy life, as well as put you on a path to health and wellness.

- *Be honest and straightforward in business and your personal life.*
- *Work with integrity and resist the temptation to sacrifice your values to "get ahead" in your profession.*
- *Never cheat, deceive, or circumvent to achieve a task.*
- *Face and accept your faults. This is honesty at its best.*
- *Try to see the good in everything and everyone. Appreciate and give thanks to those around you for who they are—even if they are imperfect.*
- *You can combine forgiveness with loving-kindness. As part of your meditation, invoke a person, incident, or event and either seek forgiveness (if you are at fault) or give forgiveness.*
- *If you perform a selfless service, silently wish that any benefit from this noble act goes to the person who needs to be forgiven. This is a double boon; in addition to being forgiven, the person also benefits from your charitable act.*
- *When you receive a lot of praises or blessings of goodwill, silently deflect the goodness to the person who needs to be forgiven.*

Reminder: For optimal results, continue to integrate the practices from all previous and future chapters into your daily routine. The more practices you can include in your life, the more results you will see!

CHAPTER 9

OVERCOMING THE DETERRENTS

"Happiness is when what you think, what you say, and what you do are in harmony."

M. K. GANDHI

Good Emotional Practices encourage the cultivation of harmonious thoughts while discarding negativity. As you work to achieve higher and higher levels of positivity, you will face emotional obstacles (or deterrents) that may prevent your progress. An inability to rid yourself of these negative traits will lead to repeated pain, suffering, dissatisfaction, and delusion.

In today's hyper-competitive world, these deterrents disrupt the body-mind-emotions nexus and overpower peace, contentment, and happiness. Sadly, it's no surprise to witness so many people, especially youngsters, suffering from poor health and inner turmoil. While the use of prescription and over-the-counter medications can mitigate some of the emotional issues and allow us to carry on with our busy lives, these quick-fix, short-term solutions prevent us from monitoring and focusing on our personal health and well-being.

Research studies suggest that individuals who display hostile and negative emotions are at risk for several chronic and inflammatory diseases. And while they don't yet fully understand how negative emotions affect the mind and body, researchers are finding that these deterrents cloud the mind and thereby cognition while also affecting the body by lowering immunity. This toxic combination results in poor health, illness, and disease.[165]

In previous chapters, you learned about the brain-gut and brain-colon nexus, as well as the importance of healthy gut and colon function as a prerequisite for a healthy brain. Your emotions play a powerful role in this as well, since stressful thoughts and negative feelings can impact the stomach and bowels. If that isn't bad enough, extended periods of chronic stress, which are characterized by heightened negativity, trigger the release of stress-associated neurochemicals that wreak havoc with the gut microbiome, digestion, and colon function.[166] This can result in a range of digestive disorders, including diarrhea, constipation, inflammatory bowel disease, and Crohn's disease, among others. Any time you experience stomach or colon issues, it is a signal to your brain that there may be a disruption in your emotional system. If you find this disruption is due to chronic stress and negative emotions, you will want to rectify these conditions as quickly as possible.

Listed below are some of the deterrents that prevent us from achieving a truly rewarding and fulfilling life. Overcoming these deterrents is a key to a peaceful life, the preservation of mental, physical, and emotional health, and ridding yourself once and for all from negativity in your life.

ANGER

In Chapter 2, verse 63, the Bhagavad Gita states: "*Anger leads to delusion which results in loss of memory. From loss of memory there is destruction of discrimination, as a result of which the individual perishes.*" According to this Eastern text, our bodies, minds, and emotions assume that worldly objects will give us pleasure and happiness. Then, by continuously thinking about these objects of desire, you create attachments to them. Attachment leads to desire, and when the desire is not fulfilled, you become angry. Anger disrupts the equilibrium between body, mind, and emotions, and leads to delusion and confusion. Eventually, this results in the failure to reason, leading to a perception that you are ruined. If nothing changes, and your life spirals out of control, what once was anger can even lead to death.

I used to wonder how the authors of these texts suspected that anger could trigger one's demise. Interestingly, evidence-based research studies report that anger stimulates hormonal and other physiological responses that are potentially life-threatening! I found even more support in the book, *Ayurvedic Secrets to Longevity & Total Health*. In this book, authors Brooks and Anselmo declare, "*When we are angry, not only do we spew out negativity to someone else, but our own body chemistry changes, and these changes can be harmful to our health."*

Likewise, other health professionals, including behavioral scientists and psychologists, agree that rage or anger is definitely hazardous to one's health. Heart researchers have clearly shown how anger contributes to coronary heart disease (CHD); anger triggers platelet activation and thrombosis, resulting in unwanted, pathological, and life-threatening blood clots. These clots can make a person more susceptible to illness, thereby lowering the immunity. As the immune system becomes compromised, pain increases, and the arteries narrow through the deposition of free fatty acids.[167]

Anger is also associated with chronic over-stimulation of the sympathetic nervous system, resulting in increased blood pressure and heart rate, and alterations of ventricular function. According to the American Heart Association and National Institute on Aging, CHD patients with higher levels of anger are more hostile and more likely to engage in CHD-risk behaviors like smoking, overeating, decreased physical activity, decreased sleep, as well as an increased use of alcohol and drugs.[168]

The Anatomy of Anger

When anger sets in, it shows up in the words spewed out by the person. Words carry strong, energetic vibrations, and pleasing sounds trigger the release of feel-good chemicals that calm the receiver and put him or her in a positive state. Words like "peace" or "I love you" can calm the body, mind, and emotions while also contributing to the healing process. Harshly worded language, on the other hand, not only stresses out the recipient but also inflicts a lot of mental and emotional pain. But it doesn't stop there, as the anger harms the person possessing this fiery emotion in the first place.

Cloaked under the umbrella of anger are other stressful emotions, including rage, envy, jealousy, judgment, and hypercriticism. These can all destabilize the synchronicity between the body, mind, and emotions. They can also exhaust one's mental and physical energy levels and lower the levels of feel-good neurochemicals and hormones.

If you or anyone you know has anger issues, it is critical to seriously consider anger management techniques. Some of these techniques include eating high-prana foods, daily mental and physical exercise, engaging in five-sense therapies, establishing good sleep habits, providing selfless service, meditating consistently, and practicing the five noble intentions regularly.

This combination of therapies will not only bring the body, mind, and emotions back in sync, but it will also help curb anger and other negative feelings. While many anger management techniques do not cure the individual, by incorporating these Good Living Practices, you—or those around you—will identify anger at its inception. As a result, the anger process will not evoke the same physical and emotional reactions, as it can be curtailed even before it rises.

ADDICTION

Addiction is the repetition of a specific behavior, practice, or action that is beyond control despite adverse consequences. People who have an addiction are enslaved to it and do not have control over what they are doing, taking, or using. I consider addiction a deterrent primarily because, along with the addiction, the person experiences emotions like fear, helplessness, shame, guilt, and depression.

Addiction culminates into a negative behavior that interferes with daily responsibilities (e.g., family, work, and/or relationships), and it can also harm the person's health and wellness. Those with an addiction become entirely dependent or preoccupied with the substance or behavior.

Sometimes, they are not even aware that their addiction is causing problems for themselves and others. Examples of addictions include (but are not limited to) smoking, drug abuse, exercise and food, digital devices, gambling, and sex.

The Bhagavad Gita reveals this truth about addiction: "*Bewildered by the sensual desires and addicted to these sensory pleasures only brings downfall to the individual.*" I believe that, along this pathway to destruction, the addicted person lives in a low-prana state. If you recall from Chapter 1, I defined prana as the vital power, energy, or force that keeps the body, mind, and emotions integrated into a single entity. Addiction destabilizes the body, mind, and emotions, creating mental and emotional turbulence, with negative repercussions on physical health.

Research reveals that addiction changes both brain structure and function.[169] While anger damages the heart, addiction destroys the brain. But it's not only substances like drugs and alcohol that co-opt certain areas of the brain; other pleasurable yet addictive activities, such as gambling, shopping, food, tech devices, and sex, can also stimulate the same neuronal network. Regardless of the activity, the brain responds in the same way— the addictive behavior triggers a powerful surge of a neurochemical called dopamine, which puts the person in a state of euphoria. This euphoric feeling creates a strong desire to continue the addictive behavior, resulting in overloading the brain with dopamine.[170] As the addiction continues through repeated exposure, it causes the nerve cells to crave more. This vicious cycle creates the conditions of tolerance and withdrawal. While tolerance is the ability of the body and mind to continually adapt to the addiction and seek larger doses to achieve the same effect, withdrawal refers to the physical, mental, and emotional symptoms that arise when reducing or abstaining from the addictive behavior.

Addiction does not fall under the purview of habit because the person is truly unable to control the process. A habit is a willful practice, engaged in by choice, and the individual is in a position to stop it, and they rarely have consequences as adverse as the consequences of addiction. The long-term penalty of addiction is a downward spiral of body-mind-emotional dysfunction, abuse, and poor health, leaving behind a trail of shame and guilt.

Those with serious addiction issues need to consider appropriate de-addiction management techniques. There are effective therapy programs, but these can be pricey. On the other hand, a self-initiated home therapy de-addiction program would include practicing everything that I have listed in the book thus far, including a high prana diet, proper eating habits, a daily regimen of controlled physical exercise, a regular five-sense maintenance program, a consistent mental exercise regimen, good sleeping habits, selfless service, meditation, and practicing the five noble intentions regularly. As with anger, this combinatorial therapy will ensure the unity of the body, mind, and emotions to alter the neural network system. Over time, this can promote higher cessation and lower relapse rates. Ultimately, these natural techniques empower people to overcome addiction and place themselves in an upward spiral of good health and wellness.

ANXIETY

Anxiety is an emotion that most of us experience at some point. It may surface while working, before taking a test, while making an important decision, or on the first day at a new job, to name just a few. While these examples are short-lived experiences that may induce anxiety, chronic anxiety is different. Chronic anxiety is generally accompanied by fear and worry. Together, these emotions generate distress. When they reach a certain level for a sustained period, they can even interfere with our ability to lead normal lives.[171]

There are many reasons why someone may suffer from anxiety; it could stem from early childhood experiences, a traumatic event, abuse, or even genetics. Regardless of the origin, chronic anxiety disrupts the delicate balance between the body, mind, and emotions. Eventually, the individual suffering from anxiety will live in a state of constant fear, nervousness, and/or obsessive-compulsive disorder. The downstream effects include both psychological and physical symptoms.[172]

Chronic anxiety triggers the flight or fight response, resulting in an increased heart rate, shortness of breath, panic, uneasiness, and muscle tension. Other symptoms include light-headedness, sleep issues, nausea, diarrhea, and frequent urination. Thus, what appears to be a simple emotion can take a serious toll on the mind and body. Recent studies have shown that chronic anxiety can also lower one's life span. In one study, researchers analyzed data from hundreds of evidence-based studies involving nearly 70,000 patients. The researchers concluded that people with anxiety might suffer from reduced life expectancies after taking into account other health and lifestyle factors. The combination of stress, poor mental and physical health, and the intake of anti-anxiety medications are responsible for these reduced lifespans.[173]

Chronic anxiety clouds the mind and ability to reason. This, in turn, leads to a disharmonious life. The great philosopher Ralph Waldo Emerson remarked, "***Nothing can bring you peace but yourself.***" While anti-anxiety medications may serve as a quick fix, it may reduce one's motivation to focus on personal health and well being. Instead, a safe, long-term, home therapy program would include practicing everything that I have already discussed (high-prana diet, mental and physical exercise, etc.). At the risk of being redundant, these various therapies not only help alleviate addictions and anger issues but also effectively treat and eliminate feelings of anxiety.

DEPRESSION

Depression is another extremely complex emotional disease, where someone experiences overwhelming sadness and loneliness—sometimes for unknown reasons. Like the previous deterrents, depression disrupts the body, mind, and emotions in all facets of life. Depression crushes peace, contentment, and happiness, resulting in poor health and suffering.

While depression prevents someone from enjoying life, its effects go far beyond mood alone, as it also impacts energy, sleep, appetite, and physical health.[174] Factors that trigger depression include but are not limited to: abuse, certain medications, personal/professional/social conflicts, loss of a loved one, chronic illness, substance abuse, some traumatic experience, or social isolation. Depression is also commonly seen in people who also have other chronic illnesses, including diabetes, cancer, obesity, memory loss, other neurodegenerative conditions, and heart disease. Depression can have serious consequences that can affect every aspect of an individual's life. Suicide, addiction, self-harm, social isolation, and relationship issues are some of the complications associated with depression.[175] Several research studies suggest that severe depression may also trigger rapid and unhealthy aging.[176]

While the use of anti-depressant medications can mitigate some of the health issues and allow the individual to carry on normally, the long-term side effects of these medications result in poor health and wellbeing. Fortunately, there is good news: all the tools described in this book allow an individual with depression to overcome this emotional condition and its associated symptoms. In fact, the following story will illustrate the power of these practices:

CASE STUDY

Alex came to me, desperate for advice and assistance after his therapist suggested he begin a regimen of anti-depressants. "I know that I'm depressed, and I need to do something, but I don't like the idea of being on medication for the rest of my life," he sighed.

"Tell me a bit about what has been going on in your life," I suggested. With that, Alex shared a complicated life history, where addiction and abuse were the norm in his home—until he was put into foster care. And although his foster family was supportive and loving, for a time, nothing could seem to fill the void in Alex's heart for love and acceptance from his biological family.

"I was kind of rough on my foster family as a teenager," he confided. "Drinking, drugs—you name it! The adrenaline high from taking risks during that period in my life probably made my foster family think I had a death wish, and maybe, in some ways, I did."

Fortunately, the loving guidance of his foster family motivated him to graduate from high school and go to college, after which he was hired as a financial advisor for a large company. Life was looking up for Alex—with a marriage on the horizon and a job promotion in his near future.

But then, things came crashing down again. The financial crisis led to layoffs, and Alex was one of them. To make matters worse, the love of his life decided she no longer wanted to get married. "Guess I was good enough when the money was coming in, but she clearly didn't love me—because as soon as I got laid off, she was out the door!"

Now, three years later, Alex was again gainfully employed, but the feelings of loss and sorrow had not lifted. "Some days, I can barely get myself out of bed. And at night, I'm noticing that my drinking has been on the rise. I can't seem to shake these feelings, but I have enough awareness to know that I can't go on like this forever. Something's got to give, and I'm afraid I'm going to head down the wrong path, like I did years ago, if I don't do something immediately. But like I said, I don't want to go on meds. What can I do?"

Because he still had enough motivation to seek out my help, I knew there was hope that he would follow through with a strict diet, exercise, and emotional wellness regimen. First, I asked him to cut out as many low-prana foods as possible in his diet and replace them with high-prana choices. He already belonged to a gym (even though he hadn't been going), so I asked him to commit to working out at least five days a week. On the days he wasn't at the gym, I asked him to walk in the woods near his house, barefoot, for proper grounding. I gave him a list of the exercises that tune the sense organs, as well as asking that he spend the first ten minutes of his day meditating.

During the day, I requested that he smile at least once every hour and suggested he set an alarm on his phone as a reminder, and before he went to bed, I wanted him to keep a gratitude journal. In it, I wanted him to focus on the positive aspects of his life—past and present, including any positive aspects of his biological family—to begin the process of forgiving his parents while recognizing all of the good things in his life. "Do this for the next four weeks, and then let's meet again."

When he returned a month later, Alex walked into my office, standing taller than the first time I met him—and with a genuine smile on his face. His eyes looked brighter, and he appeared to be taking full, cleansing breaths as he sat down.

"So," I asked, "How did it go this past month?"

He smiled once again, sharing with me all of his successes from the month: more energy, better sleep, a sense of peace and oneness after daily meditation—and even feeling less angry about his past.

"Of course, not everything's perfect. I still have moments of sadness and doubt, but I feel like something has shifted internally. In fact, I actually have hope that I can overcome this without medication!"

Alex's motivation to overcome his mental issues reminded me of Swami Sivananda's quote, "Do not brood over your past mistakes and failures as this will only fill your mind with grief, regret, and depression. Do not repeat them in the future."

GREED

In the words of Mahatma Gandhi, "*The world has enough for everyone's needs, but not enough for everyone's greed.*" That sums up the definition of greed—an emotional trait characterized by a strong desire for material possessions. It is an uncontrollable, excessive, and unappeasable longing for material benefits, including food, money, jewelry, status, or power. Greed forces people to acquire material possessions and surround themselves with them. But in the process, they lose the ability to take only what is truly necessary—and no more.

Thus, greedy people get caught up in an endless loop of acquiring or possessing materials without ever being satisfied. In the effort to possess or acquire, their mind and emotions get clouded to an extent where they may even resort to nefarious activities (scavenging, hoarding, theft, robbery, etc.) to acquire the object(s) of their desire. Greedy people consider their possessions an essential part of their identity, so losing or disposing of a possession may induce anger, extreme anxiety, a sense of loss, grief, or depression, putting them in a loop of endless negativity.[177]

Greed extinguishes positive traits like honesty and loving-kindness and replaces them with deception, envy, anger, anxiety, addiction, and depression. Over time, these emotions build up and affect the normal mindset and thinking process.[178]

Like the previous four deterrents, the easiest and most effective way to overcome greed is to introduce this book's dietary, exercise, mental, and emotional exercises into one's lifestyle. While these tools may not completely reverse this powerful negative emotion, the individual may begin to gradually navigate away from greed and move toward other, more positive emotions.

Tips from the GLP Toolbox for Deterrents

In addition to the suggestions from the previous chapters in this book, consider the following tips and tricks to overcome deterrents:

- *Avoiding meat entirely is a terrific way to jump-start a high-prana diet and experience immediate positive benefits. Meat is a low-prana food that clouds positive emotions while promoting negative ones. If you find these deterrents to be a challenge in your life, take action by avoiding meat today.*

- *If you're experiencing a surge of emotions, allow your mind and emotional state to calm down before eating.*

- *Remember to continue a daily habit of fasting between twelve and fifteen hours between dinner and breakfast. This allows your emotional state to remain in sync and resonate with your inner and outer life.*

- *In addition to its other benefits, chewing food well can help defog the mind and overcome negative emotions.*

- *Because public places, restaurants, and meeting rooms sometimes carry negative external stimuli, avoid eating in these places if you struggle with any of the deterrents.*

- *When your emotions surge, add twenty more minutes to your exercise routine.*

- *Grounding exercises are a highly effective way to overcome negative emotions. Walk on the beach barefoot, or engage in yard work without gloves. Remain focused as you engage in these activities to transform them into meditative ones.*

- *Provide a fresh meal to at least three needy people once a month. Refer to Chapter 6 for more ideas for selfless service acts.*

- *Recommit to cultivating one of the noble five intentions (contentment, honesty, loving-kindness, forgiveness, and non-violence) to overcome deterrents.*

Reminder: For optimal results, continue to integrate the practices from all previous chapters into your daily routine. The more practices you can include in your life, the more results you will see!

ACKNOWLEDGMENTS

Writing this book was more rewarding and uplifting than I could have ever imagined. It would not have been possible without the support of my awesome wife, Padma. From reading the drafts to the wonderful discussions about the Good Living Practices, Padma's support and patience were instrumental in getting this book done.

I wish to acknowledge the invaluable advice and assistance from the following people during the initial drafting and development of this book: Padma Priya, Elizabeth Savelli, Karen Poksay, Mary Thompson, Nina Zolotow, Patrice Priya Wagner, Dr. Diana Lurie, and Cathy Turney.

My research tenure at the Buck Institute for Research on Aging was outstanding in teaching me new skills, including developing professional working relationships, project planning, management and direction, supervising lab staff, communicating the results, and a strong work ethic. Therefore, I wish to express special appreciation to Dr. Dale Bredesen, laboratory colleagues, including Veena Theendakara, Alexander Patent, Clare A. Peters Libeu, Karen S. Poksay, Qiang Zhang, Patricia Spilman, Michael Ellerby, Sylvia Chen, Alyson Peel, Evan Hermel, Lisa Ellerby, Rowena Abulencia, and Molly Susag. We conducted incredible research on neurodegeneration with emphasis on Alzheimer's disease—and had fascinating discussions about aging, neurodegeneration, integrative sciences, and optimal health and wellness. This research laid the foundation for this book. I truly cherish and value their friendship.

I am grateful to Denise Kalos and her group at AFFIRMATIVhealth for their notable work on the personalized, comprehensive treatment plans for early-stage Alzheimer's disease and other forms of dementia. I was fortunate to be a consultant on this team and the research study for several months, providing help to many people with cognitive issues.

I am grateful to the following scientists for their guidance and teaching during the initial stages of my research career: Professors A.S. Balasubramanian, K.A.Balu, Stephen S. Brimijoin, Laurence J.Miller, and Anthony J. Windebank.

Thanks go as well to Dr. Marc Halpern, Director of the California College of Ayurveda, Mary Thompson, Devi Mueller, Jacob Griscom, Debra Riordan, Suzanne Ropiequet, Rob Talbert, John Allan, and the rest of the faculty and staff for supporting me on my Ayurveda journey.

I also wish to express my sincere gratitude to the numerous Yoga teachers, including Dr. Baxter Bell, Nina Zolotow, Erika Trice, Erin Fleming, Peggy Orr, Maritza, Nikki Estrada, Michele Klink, Richard Rosen, and others from whom I learned the best of Yoga and Yoga philosophy.

A heartfelt thanks to all my Ayurveda patients for entrusting me with your care. My successful journey of Ayurveda was made possible thanks to your confidence and trust in me. It is a real privilege to have the opportunity of recommending these Good Living Practices and seeing you all get better and leading a high quality and optimal life.

Special thanks and words of appreciation to all my students of Yoga and Ayurveda for trusting me as your guide as you went through your learning. Please remember that each one of you was a teacher to me. I gained a lot of learning from you as much as you allowed me to teach you.

My respect and appreciation also go to Master Stephen Co, Chandan Parmeswara, and all other practitioners of Pranic Healing. My journey into the world of Pranic Healing helped me to understand and appreciate the infinite source of energy we have access to and utilize this energy to nourish and stabilize our body, mind, and emotions.

For the numerous discussions over the years about various concepts from the Vedic texts, including the cosmos, life on earth, the three aspects of individuality, and human health and wellness, my profound thanks to Kumar Padmini and all members of the Satsang group.

Finally, I wish to express my heartfelt thanks and appreciation to Howard VanEs and his team at Let's Write Books, Inc. for guiding me through the publishing process and helping create a book that exceeded my expectations.

ABOUT RAMMOHAN RAO, PhD

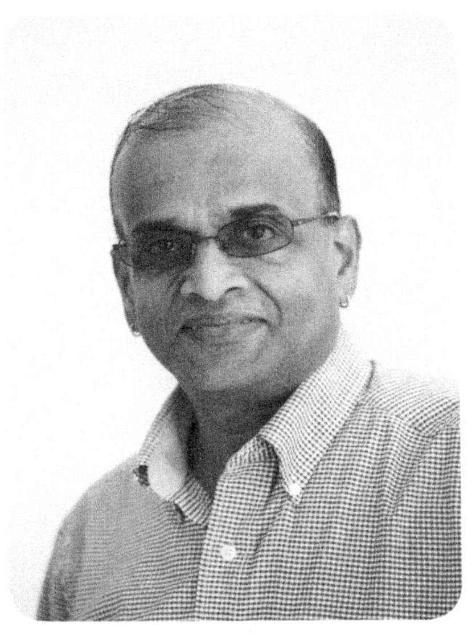

Rammohan Rao (Ram) is passionate about helping people live vibrant, healthy, and purposed-filled lives through natural methods and has dedicated his life to the research and integration of modern science with Eastern practices.

Ram holds a PhD in neuroscience and was a research associate professor of neuroscience at the Buck Institute for Research on Aging, Novato, CA. His research focused on chronic stress, neuronal cell death, and mechanisms of age-associated neurodegenerative diseases, with special emphasis on Alzheimer's disease. Ram has over twenty years of research and teaching experience in neuroscience and has published more than fifty peer-reviewed papers in scientific journals, including chapters in several textbooks.

Ram is also a NAMA Board Certified Ayurveda Practitioner (AP), a Registered Yoga Teacher (RYT-200), and he teaches Ayurveda and Yoga at the California College of Ayurveda. Ram has published several articles in major Yoga/Ayurveda magazines and has been a featured speaker in several national and international meetings and symposia on Yoga & Ayurveda. Ram is a member of the NAMA Accreditation Committee and Editor of Ayurveda Journal of Health.

In his spare time, he offers consultations in YAMP techniques (Yoga, Ayurveda, Meditation, and Pranayama), and conducts YAMP workshops, seminars, and cooking classes. Ram's passion for serving others and teaching has also led him to mentor high school students, college interns, research technicians, and post-doctoral fellows. To learn more about Ram, visit:

1. **KaivalyaWellness.com**
2. **Yoga for Healthy Aging:** www.yogaforhealthyaging.blogspot.com/search/label/Ram%20Rao

   (This site has more than 100 articles written by Ram on yoga, health, and wellness.)

3. **Accessible Yoga Blog:** www.accessibleyoga.blogspot.com/search/label/Ram%20Rao

   (Ram is one of the contributing members and regularly posts articles on yoga, health, and wellness.)

4. **Facebook:** www.facebook.com/ram.rao.351?ref=bookmarks

   (Ram regularly posts interesting blurbs on neuroscience, yoga, Ayurveda, health, and wellness.)

5. **California College of Ayurveda:** www.ayurvedacollege.com/college/ayurveda-faculty

   (Check this site for Ram's teaching schedule, classes, and workshops)

ENDNOTES

CHAPTER 1

1 *The Vedic texts* are a large body of religious texts written in Sanskrit and originating in ancient India. Considered as personal revelations gained from intense meditation practices by Rishis (sages and seers), these texts are a collection of hymns, poems, prayers, formulas, and other religious material that seek to understand the cosmos, the universal laws, life on earth, human life, and the connection of the earthly forms to the universe. Embedded in these texts are also concepts regarding health and wellness.

2 Rao RV. *Ayurveda and the Science of Aging*. Journal of Ayurveda and Integrative Medicine. 2018, 9(3):225-232.

3 Laska, MN et al. *How we eat what we eat: identifying meal routines and practices most strongly associated with healthy and unhealthy dietary factors among young adults*. Public Health Nutr. 2015, 18(12), 2135-45; Rao RV. *Ayurveda and the Science of Aging*. Journal of Ayurveda and Integrative Medicine. 2018, 9(3):225-232.

4 Domingo JL & Nadal M. *Carcinogenicity of consumption of red meat and processed meat: A review of scientific news since the IARC decision*. Food Chem Toxicol. 2017. 105:256-261; World Health Organization. *Carcinogenicity of the consumption of red meat and processed meat*. https://www.who.int/features/qa/cancer-red-meat/en/.

5 Grandin T. *The Effect of Stress on Livestock and Meat Quality Prior to and During Slaughter*. International Journal for the Study of Animal Problems. 1980, 1(5): 313-337.

6 Pan A et al. *Red Meat Consumption and Mortality: Results from Two Prospective Cohort Studies*. Arch Intern Med. 2012, 172(7): 555-563; Micha, R et al. *Red and processed meat consumption and risk of incident coronary heart disease, stroke, and diabetes mellitus: A systematic review and meta-analysis*. Circulation. 2010. 121(21):2271-2283.

7 Thakkar J et al. *Ritucharya: Answer to the lifestyle disorders*. Ayu. 2011. 32(4): 466-471.

8 Mohammad Asif. *Physico-chemical properties and toxic effect of fruit-ripening agent calcium carbide*. Annals of Tropical Medicine and Public health.2012. 5(3)150-156.

9 Rao RV. *Ayurveda and the Science of Aging*. Journal of Ayurveda and Integrative Medicine. 2018, 9(3):225-232.

10 Lolla A. *Mantras Help the General Psychological Well-Being of College Students: A Pilot Study*. J Relig Health. 2018. 57(1):110-119; Simon R et al. *Mantra Meditation Suppression of Default Mode Beyond an Active Task: a Pilot Study*. J Cogn Enhanc. 2017. 1:219–227.

11 Rao RV. *Ayurveda and the Science of Aging*. Journal of Ayurveda and Integrative Medicine. 2018, 9(3):225-232. Garaulet, M et al. *Timing of food intake predicts weight loss effectiveness*. Int J Obes (Lond). 2013.37(4), 604-611.

12 Murphy T et al. *Effects of Diet on Brain Plasticity in Animal and Human Studies: Mind the Gap*. Neural Plast. 2014. 1-32.

13 Alirezaei et al. *Short-term fasting induces profound neuronal autophagy*. Autophagy. 2010. 6(6): 702-710.

14 Hamada etal. *The Number of Chews and Meal Duration Affect Diet-Induced Thermogenesis and Splanchnic Circulation*. OBESITY. (2014). 22:E62–E69.

15 Tada A & Miura H. *Association between mastication and cognitive status: A systematic review*. Arch Gerontol Geriatr. 2017. 70:44-53.

16 Reynolds, KA et al. *Occurrence of bacteria* and biochemical markers on *public surfaces*. Int J Environ Health Res. 2005. 15(3):225-34; Lax S et al. *Forensic analysis of the microbiome of phones and shoes*. Microbiome. 2015. 3:21-29.

CHAPTER 2

17 McPhee JS et al. *Physical activity in older age: perspectives for healthy ageing and frailty*. Biogerontology. 2016. 17:567–580.

18 U.S. National Library of Medicine. *Benefits of exercise*. https://medlineplus.gov/benefitsofexercise.html.

19 Yuan Y et al. *The roles of exercise* in *bone* remodeling and in prevention and treatment of osteoporosis. Prog Biophys Mol Biol. 2016. 122(2):122-130.

20 Ekelund U et al. *Does physical activity* attenuate, or even eliminate, the detrimental association of sitting time with mortality? A harmonised meta-analysis of data from more than 1 million men and women. Lancet. 2016. 388(10051):1302-1310; Patel AV et al. *Leisure time spent sitting in relation to total mortality in a prospective cohort of US adults*. Am J Epidemiol. 2010.172(4):419-429.

21 Siddarth P et al. *Sedentary behavior associated with reduced medial temporal lobe thickness in middle aged and older adults*. PLoS One. 2018. 12;13(4).

22 US News & World Report. *Excessive Sitting Cuts Life Expectancy by Two Years*. https://www.usnews.com/news/articles/2012/07/09/study-excessive-sitting-cuts-life-expectancy-by-two-years.

23 *Sit, stand, sit: The new science about how to best use your standing desk*. https://www.cnn.com/2019/09/12/health/standing-desks-tips-myths-facts-wellness/index.html.

24 Harvard School of Public Health. *Obesity Prevention Source- Physical Activity*. https://www.hsph.harvard.edu/obesity-prevention-source/obesity-causes/physical-activity-and-obesity/.

25 Lee IM, et al. *Physical Activity and Weight Gain Prevention. JAMA*.2010. 303:1173-1179.

26 Wareham NJ, et al. *Physical activity and obesity prevention: a review of the current evidence. Proc Nutr Soc*. 2005. 64:229-247.

27 National Heart, Lung and Blood Institute. *Physical Activity and Your Heart*. https://www.nhlbi.nih.gov/health-topics/physical-activity-and-your-heart.

28 Colbery SR et al. *Physical Activity/Exercise and Diabetes: A Position Statement of the American Diabetes Association*. Diabetes Care. 2016. 39:2065-2079.

29 National Institute of Child Health and human development. *How does physical activity help build healthy bones*? https://www.nichd.nih.gov/health/topics/bonehealth/conditioninfo/activity.

30 Johns Hopkins School of Medicine. *Exercising for Better Sleep*. https://www.hopkinsmedicine.org/health/wellness-and-prevention/exercising-for-better-sleep.

31 Medical news Today. *Exercise may increase lifespan 'regardless of past activity levels'*. https://www.medicalnewstoday.com/articles/325610.php#1.

32 Rachael Rettner. *How Exercise Fights Inflammation*. LiveScience. https://www.livescience.com/59988-exercise-fights-inflammation.html.

33 Morgan JA et al. *Effects of physical exercise on central nervous system functions: a review of brain region specific adaptations*. Journal of Molecular Psychiatry. 2015. 3(3): 1-13.

34 Scientific American-MIND.*Why Do I Think Better after I Exercise*? https://www.scientificamerican.com/article/why-do-you-think-better-after-walk-exercise/.

35 Liu PZ & Nusslock, R. *Exercise-Mediated Neurogenesis in the Hippocampus via BDNF* Front Neurosci. 2018;12(52): 1-6.

36 Dougherty RJ et al. *Meeting physical activity recommendations may be protective against temporal lobe atrophy in older adults at risk for Alzheimer's disease.* Alzheimer's & Dementia. 2016. 4: 14-17.

37 Erickson KI et al. *Exercise training increases size of hippocampus and improves memory.* Proc Natl Acad Sci U S A. 2011. 108(7):3017-3022.

38 Morgan JA et al. *Effects of physical exercise on central nervous system functions: a review of brain region specific adaptations.* Journal of Molecular Psychiatry. 2015. 3(3):1-13.

39 Exercise Boosts Life Expectancy, Study Finds. https://www.livescience.com/news; Exercise: 7 benefits of regular physical activity. https://www.mayoclinic.org/healthy-lifestyle/fitness/in-depth/exercise/art-20048389.

40 Hurley, M. et al. *Exercise interventions and patient beliefs for people with hip, knee or hip and knee osteoarthritis: a mixed methods review.* Cochrane Database Syst Rev. 2018. 1-167.

41 Physical Activity Guidelines for Americans. https://health.gov/dietaryguidelines/2015/guidelines/appendix-1/.

42 Jaspers RT et al. *Exercise, fasting, and mimetics: toward beneficial combinations?* FASEB J. 2017. 31(1):14-28.

43 Oschman JL, et al. *The effects of grounding (earthing) on inflammation, the immune response, wound healing, and prevention and treatment of chronic inflammatory and autoimmune diseases.* Journal of Inflammation Research 2015.8: 83–96.

CHAPTER 3

44 Farahani PV et al. *Effectiveness of super brain yoga for children with hyperactivity disorder.* Perspect Psychiatr Care. 2019. 55(2):140-146.

45 Meehan, M & Penckofer, S. *The Role of Vitamin D in the Aging Adult.* J Aging Gerontol. 2014. 2(2): 60-71.

46 Mostafa, WZ & Hegazy, RA. *Vitamin D and the skin: Focus on a complex relationship: A review.* Journal of Advanced Research.2015. 6: 793-804.

47 *Science of vision: How do our eyes enable us to see*? SCIENCE. 21/09/2015. https://www.howitworksdaily.com/science-of-vision-how-do-our-eyes-enable-us-to-see/.

48 *A Good Night's Sleep*. National Institute on Aging. https://www.nia.nih.gov/health/good-nights-sleep.

49 Hannerz J. *Systemic symptoms associated with orbital venous vasculitis*. Cephalalgia.1988.8(4):255-263.

50 *Does our emotional state affect our vision*? https://visioneyeinstitute.com.au/eyematters/emotional-state-affect-vision/.

51 *Caring for Your Vision*. American Optometric Association. https://www.aoa.org/patients-and-public/caring-for-your-vision/protecting-your-vision/computer-vision-syndrome.

52 Stinton, N et al. *Influence of smell loss on taste function*. Behav Neurosci. 2010. 124(2): 256-264.

53 Pires, A et al. *Intranasal drug delivery: how, why and what for*? J Pharm Pharm Sci. 2009. 12(3): 288-311.

54 Stinton, N et al. *Influence of smell loss on taste function*. Behav Neurosci. 2010. 124(2): 256-264.

55 Messadi DV. *Oral and nonoral sources of halitosis*. J Calif Dent Assoc. 1997. 25(2):127-131.

56 Danser MM. *Tongue coating and tongue brushing: a literature review*. Int J Dent Hyg. 2003. 1(3):151-158.

57 Shanbhag VK. *Oil pulling for maintaining oral hygiene* - A review. Tradit Complement Med. 2017. 7(1):106-109.

CHAPTER 4

58 Muehsam, D et al. *The embodied mind: A review on functional genomic and neurological correlates of mind-body therapies*. Neurosci Biobehav Rev. 2017. 73:165-181.

59 Green, CS & Bavelier, D. *Exercising Your Brain: A Review of Human Brain Plasticity and Training-Induced Learning*. Psychol Aging. 2008. 23(4): 692-701.

60 Schaefer, N et al. *The malleable brain: plasticity of neural circuits and behavior - a review from students to students.* J Neurochem. 2017. 142(6):790-811.

61 Shaffer, J. *Neuroplasticity and Clinical Practice: Building Brain Power for Health.* Front Psychol. 2016. 7(1118) 1-12.

62 Bavelier, D et al. *Brain plasticity through the life span: learning to learn and action video games.* Annual review of Neuroscience. 2012. 35: 395-416.

63 Stuchlik, A. *Dynamic learning and memory, synaptic plasticity and neurogenesis: an update.* Front Behav Neurosci. 2014. 8(106):1-6.

64 Peters, R. *Ageing and the brain.* Postgrad Med J. 2006. 82(964): 84-88.

65 Gheysen F et al. *Physical activity to improve cognition in older adults: can physical activity programs enriched with cognitive challenges enhance the effects? A systematic review and meta-analysis.* Int J Behav Nutr Phys Act. 2018. 15(1):63.

66 de Lange AG et al. *The effects of memory training on behavioral and microstructural plasticity* in young and older *adults.* Hum Brain Mapp. 2017. 8(11):5666-5680; Green, CS & Bavelier, D. *Exercising Your Brain: A Review of Human Brain Plasticity and Training-Induced Learning.* Psychol Aging. 2008. 23(4): 692-701.

67 Tom Michael. *What is The Knowledge taxi test and why is the exam taken by London's black cab drivers so tough.* 2017. 18:36. https://www.thesun.co.uk/news/3307245/the-knowledge-taxi-test-london-black-cab-drivers-exam/.

68 Maguire, EA et al. *London taxi drivers and bus drivers: a structural MRI and neuropsychological analysis.* Hippocampus. 2006. 16(12): 1091-1101.

69 Ricker TJ et al.*Working memory consolidation: insights from studies on attention and working memory.* Ann N Y Acad Sci. 2018. 24(1):8-18.

70 Lithfous S et al. *Spatial* navigation in normal aging and the prodromal stage of Alzheimer's disease: insights from imaging and behavioral studies. Ageing Res Rev. 2013. 12(1):201-213.

71 Shams L& Seitz AR. *Benefits* of *multisensory learning.* Trends Cogn Sci. 2008. 12(11):411-417.

72 Teichert M & Bolz J. *How Senses Work Together: Cross-Modal Interactions between Primary Sensory Cortices.* Neural Plast. 2018. 17:1-11.

73 Wingfield A & Peelle JE. *How does hearing loss affect* the *brain?* Aging health. 2012. 8(2):107-109.

74 Gurgel, RK et al. *Relationship of Hearing loss and Dementia: a Prospective, Population-based Study.* Otol Neurotol. 2014. 35(5): 775-781.

75 *Harvard Women's Health Watch. Recognizing the mind-skin connection.* 2006. https://www.health.harvard.edu/newsletter_article/Recognizing_the_mind-skin_connection.

76 Chen Y & Lyga J. *Brain-skin connection: stress, inflammation and skin aging.* Inflamm Allergy Drug Targets. 2014. 13(3):177-190.

77 Zheng, DD et al. *Longitudinal Associations Between Visual Impairment and Cognitive Functioning: The Salisbury Eye Evaluation Study.* JAMA Ophthalmol. 2018. 136(9): 989-995.

78 Doty RL & Hawkes CH. *Chemosensory dysfunction in neurodegenerative diseases.* Handb Clin Neurol. 2019. 164:325-360.

79 Marin C et al. *Olfactory Dysfunction in Neurodegenerative Diseases.* Curr Allergy Asthma Rep. 2018. 18(8):42.

80 Rahayel, S et al. *The effect of Alzheimer's disease and Parkinson's disease on olfaction: a meta-analysis.* Behav Brain Res. 2012. 231(1):60-74.

81 Erickson KI et al. *Exercise training increases size of hippocampus and improves memory.* Proc Natl Acad Sci U S A. 2011. 108(7):3017-3022; Morgan JA et al. *Effects of physical exercise on central nervous system functions: a review of brain region specific adaptations.* Journal of Molecular Psychiatry. 2015. 3(3):1-13.

82 Tarumi, T & Zhang, R. *Cerebral blood flow in normal aging adults: cardiovascular determinants, clinical implications, and aerobic fitness.* J. Neurochemistry. 2018.144(5):595-608.

83 *Why Do I Think Better after I Exercise*? Scientific American-MIND. https://www.scientificamerican.com/article/why-do-you-think-better-after-walk-exercise/.

84 Yalcin,G & Yalcin,A. *Metabolic Syndrome and Neurodegenerative Diseases.* J Geriatr Med Gerontol. 2018, 4(042):1-3.

85 Lu,B. et al. *BDNF and synaptic plasticity, cognitive function, and dysfunction.* Handb Exp Pharmacol. 2014;220:223-250.

86 Liu, PZ & Nusslock,R.. *Exercise-Mediated Neurogenesis in the Hippocampus via BDNF* Front Neurosci. 2018;12(52): 1-6.

87 Zhang Y, et al. *The Effects of Mind-Body Exercise on Cognitive Performance in Elderly: A Systematic Review and Meta-Analysis.* Int J Environ Res Public Health. 2018. 15(12):1-16.

88 Rousseaud A et al. *Bone-brain crosstalk and potential associated diseases.* Horm Mol Biol Clin Investig. 2016. 28(2):69-83.

89 Jones, KB et al. *Bone and Brain. A Review of Neural, Hormonal, and Musculoskeletal Connections.* Iowa Orthop J. 2004.24:123–132.

90 Kelly, RR et al. *Impacts of Psychological Stress on Osteoporosis: Clinical Implications and Treatment Interactions.* Front. Psychiatry. 2019.10 (200): 1-21.

91 Rousseaud A et al. Bone-brain crosstalk and potential associated diseases. Horm Mol Biol Clin Investig. 2016. 28(2):69-83; Jones, KB et al. *Bone and Brain. A Review of Neural, Hormonal, and Musculoskeletal Connections.* Iowa Orthop J. 2004.24:123–132; Kelly, RR et al. *Impacts of Psychological Stress on Osteoporosis: Clinical Implications and Treatment Interactions.* Front. Psychiatry. 2019.10 (200): 1-21.

92 Shan C et al. *Roles* for *osteocalcin* in *brain signalling: implications* in *cognition- and motor-related disorders.* Mol Brain. 2019 12(1):23-34.

93 Park MN etal. *The relationship between primary headache and constipation in children and adolescents.* Korean J Pediatr. 2015. 58(2):60-63.

94 Portalatin M et al. *Medical Management of Constipation.* Clinics in Colon and Rectal Surgery. 2012.25:12–19.

95 Furness JB & Stebbing MJ. *The first brain: Species comparisons and evolutionary implications for the enteric and central nervous systems.* Neurogastroenterol Motil. 2018. 30(2):13234.

96 Nall R. *How is stress linked with constipation.* Medical News Today. 2019. https://www.medicalnewstoday.com/articles/326970.php.

97 Chang YM et al. *Does stress induce bowel dysfunction*? Expert Rev Gastroenterol Hepatol. 2014. 8(6):583-585.

98 Dossett, M. *Brain-gut connection explains why integrative treatments can help relieve digestive ailments.* Harvard Health Blog. 2019. https://www.health.harvard.edu/blog/brain-gut-connection-explains-why-integrative-treatments-can-help-relieve-digestive-ailments-2019041116411.

99 Miller, I. *The gut–brain axis: historical reflections.* Microb Ecol Health Dis. 2018; 29(1): 1-8.

100 Fung, TC et al. *Interactions between the microbiota, immune and nervous systems in health and disease.* Nat Neurosci. 2017. 20(2):145-155.

101 Dossett, M. *Brain-gut connection explains why integrative treatments can help relieve digestive ailments.* Harvard Health Blog. 2019. https://www.health.harvard.edu/blog/brain-gut-connection-explains-why-integrative-treatments-can-help-relieve-digestive-ailments-2019041116411; Miller, I. *The gut–brain axis: historical reflections.* Microb Ecol Health Dis. 2018; 29(1): 1-8.; Fung, TC et al. *Interactions between the microbiota, immune and nervous systems in health and disease.* Nat Neurosci. 2017. 20(2):145-155.

CHAPTER 5

102 Medic, G et al. *Short- and long-term health consequences of sleep disruption.* Nature and Science of Sleep. 2017. 9:151–161.

103 *Importance of Sleep: Six reasons not to scrimp on sleep.* Harvard Health Publishing. https://www.health.harvard.edu/press_releases/importance_of_sleep_and_health.

104 Benveniste, H. *The Brain's Waste-Removal System.* Cerebrum. 2018.1-12.

105 Colten HR & Altevogt BM. *Extent and Health Consequences of Chronic Sleep Loss and Sleep Disorders. Sleep Disorders and Sleep Deprivation: An Unmet Public Health Problem.* 2006. Ch:3. 55-135. https://www.ncbi.nlm.nih.gov/books/NBK19961/.

106 Rasch B & Born J. *About sleep's role* in *memory.* Physiol Rev. 2013. 93(2):681-766.

107 Pillai JA & Leverenz JB. *Sleep* and *Neurodegeneration: A Critical Appraisal.* Chest. 2017. 151(6):1375-1386.

108 Medic, G. et al. *Short- and long-term health consequences of sleep disruption.* Nat Sci Sleep. 2017. 9:151-161.

109 Gillin, JC et al. *Sleep Aids and Insomnia.* National Sleep Foundation. https://www.sleepfoundation.org/articles/sleep-aids-and-insomnia.

110 *Sleeping Pills*: A Global Strategic Business Report. 2018. https://www.prweb.com/releases/sleeping_pills/sleeping_tablets/prweb4318034.htm.

111 Carr, T. *The Problem With Sleeping Pills*. December 12, 2018. https://www.consumer-reports.org/drugs/the-problem-with-sleeping-pills/.

112 Mayo Clinic Staff. *Prescription sleeping pills: What's right for you*? Jan 30, 2018. https://www.mayoclinic.org/diseases-conditions/insomnia/in-depth/sleeping-pills/art-20043959.

113 Finan, PH et al. *The Effects of Sleep Continuity Disruption on Positive Mood and Sleep Architecture in Healthy Adults*. SLEEP. 2015. 38(11):1735-1742.

114 Dinges, D. et al., *Cumulative Sleepiness, Mood Disturbance, and Psychomotor Vigilance Decrements During a Week of Sleep Restricted to 4 – 5 Hours Per Night*. SLEEP. 1997. 20 (4):267–277.

115 Kitamura S. et al. *Estimating individual optimal sleep duration and potential sleep debt*. Sci Rep. 2016.24(6):35812.

116 Voiss, P. et al. *The use of mind-body medicine among US individuals with sleep problems: analysis of the 2017 National Health Interview Survey data*. Sleep Medicine. 2019. 56:151-156.

117 Cordi, MJ et al. *Effects of Relaxing Music on Healthy Sleep*. Scientific Reports. 2019. 9(1):9079-9087.

CHAPTER 6

118 Konrath, S. *Motives for volunteering are associated with mortality risk in older adults*. Health Psychol. 2012. 31(1):87-96.

119 Dossey, L. *The Helper's High*. EXPLORE. 2018. 14:393-399.

120 Dambrun, M. *Self-centeredness and selflessness: happiness correlates and mediating psychological processes*. PeerJ. 2017, 5:1-27.

121 Konrath, S. *Motives* for *volunteering* are *associated* with *mortality risk* in *older adults*. Health Psychol. 2012. 31(1):87-96; Dossey, L. *The Helper's High*. EXPLORE. 2018. 14:393-399.

122 Oman, D, et al. *Volunteerism and Mortality among the Community-dwelling Elderly*. J Health Psychol. 1999. 4(3):301-316.

123 Ritvo, E. *The Neuroscience of Giving*. Psychology Today. 2014. https://www.psychologytoday.com/us/blog/vitality/201404/the-neuroscience-giving.

124 Renter, E. *What Generosity Does to Your Brain and Life Expectancy.* HEALTH. U.S. News & World Report.2015.

125 Post, SG. *It's good to be good: science says it's so. Research demonstrates that people who help others usually have healthier, happier lives.* Health Prog. 2009 90(4):18-25.

126 Ritvo, E. *The Neuroscience of Giving*. Psychology Today. 2014. https://www psychologytoday.com/us/blog/vitality/201404/the-neuroscience-giving; Renter, E. *What Generosity Does to Your Brain and Life Expectancy.* HEALTH. U.S. News & World Report.2015; Post, SG. *It's good to be good: science says it's so. Research demonstrates that people who help others usually have healthier, happier lives.* Health Prog. 2009 90(4):18-25.

127 Post, SG. *Altuism, happiness, and health: it's good to be good.* International Journal of Behavioral Medicine. 2005.12(2): 66–77.

128 Gormley, KJ. *Altruism: a framework for caring and providing care.* International Journal of Nursing Studies. 1996. 33(6), 581-588; University of California - Los Angeles. *Your brain might be hard-wired for altruism: Neuroscience research suggests an avenue for treating the empathically challenged.* ScienceDaily, 18 March 2016. http://www.sciencedaily.com/releases/2016/03/160318102101.htm.

129 Iyengar, BKS. Light on Yoga: The Bible of Modern Yoga. Paperback–January 3, 1995.

CHAPTER 7

130 Mihaly Csikszentmihalyi. *Flow: The Psychology of Optimal Experience.* 2008.

131 *Meditation: In Depth.* National Center for Complimentary and Integrative Health. https://nccih.nih.gov/health/meditation/overview.htm.

132 Wells, R. E. et al. *Meditation's impact on default mode network and hippocampus in mild cognitive impairment: a pilot study.* Neurosci Lett. 2013. 556:15-19; Tolahunase, M. R. et al. *Yoga- and meditation-based lifestyle intervention increases neuroplasticity and reduces severity of major depressive disorder: A randomized controlled trial.* Restor Neurol Neurosci.2018.36(3):423-442; Christie, G. J. et al. *Do Lifestyle Activities Protect Against Cognitive Decline in Aging? A Review.* Front Aging Neurosci. 2017. 9:381-393.

133 Peters, R. *Ageing and the brain.* Postgrad Med J. 2006. 82:84–88.

134 Luders, E. et al. *Forever Young(er): potential age-defying effects of long-term meditation on gray matter atrophy*. Front Psychol. 2015. 5:1-7.

135 Newberg, A. B. et al. *Meditation effects on cognitive function and cerebral blood flow in subjects with memory loss: a preliminary study*. Journal of Alzheimer's disease. 2010. 20(2):517-526.

136 *Meditation: In Depth*. National Center for Complimentary and Integrative Health. https://nccih.nih.gov/health/meditation/overview.htm.

137 *With mindfulness, life's in the moment*. HEALTH & MEDICINE. The Harvard Gazette. https://news.harvard.edu/gazette/story/2018/04/less-stress-clearer-thoughts-with-mindfulness-meditation/; Wegela, K.K. *How to Practice Mindfulness Meditation*. Psychology Today. https://www.psychologytoday.com/us/blog/the-courage-be-present/201001/how-practice-mindfulness-meditation.

138 Transcendental meditation. The technique for inner peace and wellness. https://www.tm.org.

139 Beginner's Body Scan Meditation. Mindful-healthy mind, healthy life. https://www.mindful.org/beginners-body-scan-meditation/.

140 Passage Meditation: The Basics. Make Your Life a Work of Art. Blue Mountain Center of Meditation. https://www.bmcm.org/about/.

141 Swami Sitaramananda. *What is Yoga Meditation? https://sivanandayogafarm.org;* Raja Yoga Meditation. https://www.brahmakumaris.org/meditation/raja-yoga-meditation.

142 World Pranic Healing Foundation. https://www.worldpranichealing.com/en/twin-hearts-meditation-benefits; https://www.globalpranichealing.com/pranic-healing/meditation-on-twin-hearts

CHAPTER 8

143 Tugade, MM. et al. *Psychological resilience and positive emotional granularity: examining the benefits of positive emotions on coping and health*. Journal of Personality. 2004. 72(6):1161–1190.

144 Lyubomirsky, S. et al. *The benefits of frequent positive affect: Does happiness lead to success? Psychological Bulletin*. 2005.131(6):803-855.

145 Diener, E. & Chan, MY. *Happy people live longer: Subjective well-being contributes to health and longevity*. Applied Psychology: Health and Well-Being. 2011.3(1):1-43

146 Kraft TL, & Pressman SD. *Grin and bear it: the influence of manipulated facial expression on the* stress response. Psychol Sci. 2012. 23(11):1372-1378; Lyubomirsky, S. et al. *The benefits of frequent positive affect: Does happiness lead to success? Psychological Bulletin*. 2005.131(6):803-855; Diener, E. & Chan, MY. *Happy people live longer: Subjective well-being contributes to health and longevity*. Applied Psychology: Health and Well-Being. 2011.3(1):1-43.

147 Korb, A. *The Grateful Brain. The neuroscience of giving thanks*. Psychology Today. 2012 https://www.psychologytoday.com/us/blog/prefrontal-nudity/201211/the-grateful-brain.

148 Sansone,RA & Sansone, LA. *Gratitude and Well Being. The Benefits of Appreciation*. Psychiatry (Edgmont). 2010.7(11):18–22.

149 Zahn, R. et al. *The Neural Basis of Human Social Values: Evidence from Functional MRI* Cereb Cortex. 2009 Feb; 19(2): 276–283.

150 Luskin, F. *The art and science of forgiveness*. Stanford Medicine. 1999. 16(4). http://sm.stanford.edu/archive/stanmed/1999summer/forgiveness.html.

151 Mayo Clinic Staff. *Forgiveness: Letting go of grudges and bitterness*. Healthy Lifestyle-Adult health. https://www.mayoclinic.org/healthy-lifestyle/adult-health/in-depth/forgiveness/art-20047692.

152 Toussaint, LL. et al. *Forgive to Live: Forgiveness, Health, and Longevity*. Journal of Behavioral Medicine. 2012.35(4):375-386.

153 vanOyen,WC. et al. *Granting forgiveness or harboring grudges: Implications for emotions, physiology, and health*. Psychological Science. 2001.12(2):117-123.

154 American Psychological Association. *Lying Less Linked to Better Health, New Research Finds*. https://www.apa.org/news/press/releases/2012/08/lying-less.

155 Iliades, C. *The Truth About Lies*. Everyday Health. 2010. July 14. https://www.everydayhealth.com/longevity/truth-about-lies-and-longevity.aspx; Mayo Clinic Staff. *Chronic stress puts your health at risk*. Healthy Lifestyle-Stress management https://www.mayoclinic.org/healthy-lifestyle/stress-management/in-depth/stress/art-20046037.

156 Dike, CC. *Pathological lying: symptom or disease*. 2008. http://www.psychiatrictimes.com/articles/pathological-lying-symptom-or-disease.

157 Pace TW. et al. *Effect of compassion meditation on neuroendocrine, innate immune and behavioral responses to psychosocial stress*. Psychoneuroendocrinology. 2009.34(1):87-98.

158 Lutz A. et al. *Regulation of the neural circuitry of emotion by compassion meditation: effects of meditative expertise.* PLoS One. 2008.3(3). e1897.

159 CBS News Report: *U.S. life expectancy lowest among wealthy nations due to disease, violence.* 2013. https://www.cbsnews.com/news/report-us-life-expectancy-lowest-among-wealthy-nations-due-to-disease-violence/.

160 Rutherford. A. et al. *Violence: a glossary.* J Epidemiol & Community Health. 2007. 61(8):676–680.

161 Siever, LJ. *Neurobiology of Aggression and Violence.* Am J Psychiatry. 2008.165(4):429-442; Rivara, F et al. *The Effects Of Violence On Health.* HealthAffairs. 2019.38(10):1622-1629.

162 Springer, KW et al. *The long-term health outcomes of childhood abuse. An overview and a call to action.* J Gen Intern Med. 2003.18(10):864-870.

163 The National Coalition Against Domestic Violence (NCADV)-RESOURCES. https://ncadv.org/resources; M.K. Gandhi Institute for Nonviolence. https://gandhiinstitute.org/mission-history/; FUTURES Without Violence. https://www.futureswithoutviolence.org/our-mission/; The Martin Luther King, Jr. Center for Nonviolent Social Change. https://thekingcenter.org/about-king-center/.

164 Tugade, MM. et al. *Psychological resilience and positive emotional granularity: examining the benefits of positive emotions on coping and health.* Journal of Personality. 2004. 72(6):1161–1190.

CHAPTER 9

165 Du J, Huang J, An Y, Xu W. *The relationship between stress and negative emotion: The Mediating role of rumination.* Clin Res Trials. 2018.4(1):1-5; Charles,ST et al. *The Wear and Tear of Daily Stressors on Mental Health.* Psychological Science, 2013.24(5):733-741.

166 Pogosyan,M. *Are Negative Emotions Universally Bad for Our Health*? Psychology Today. 2019. https://www.psychologytoday.com/us/blog/between-cultures/201906/are-negative-emotions-universally-bad-our-health.

167 Staicu,M-L & Cutov, M. *Anger and health risk behaviors.* Journal of Medicine and Life.2010.3(4):372-375; *Anger-how it affects people.* Better Health Channel. Victoria State Government. https://www.betterhealth.vic.gov.au/health/healthyliving/anger-how-it-affects-people.

168 Kawachi, I et al. *A Prospective Study of Anger and Coronary Heart Disease*-The Normative Aging Study. Circulation.1996.94:2090–2095; *Coping with Feelings.* American Heart Association. https://www.heart.org/en/health-topics/cardiac-rehab/taking-care-of-yourself/coping-with-feelings.

169 Harvard Mental Health Letter. *How addiction hijacks the brain.* Harvard Health Publishing. July 2011. https://www.health.harvard.edu/newsletter_article/how-addiction-hijacks-the-brain.

170 NIH News in Health. *Biology of Addiction-Drugs and Alcohol Can Hijack Your Brain.* October 2015. https://newsinhealth.nih.gov/2015/10/biology-addiction.

171 Harvard Women's Health Watch. *Anxiety and physical illness.* Harvard Health Publishing. May 2018. https://www.health.harvard.edu/staying-healthy/anxiety_and_physical_illness.

172 National Institute of Mental Health. *Anxiety Disorders.* https://www.nimh.nih.gov/health/topics/anxiety-disorders/index.shtml.

173 ScienceDaily. *Poor mental health linked to reduced life expectancy.* July 2012. https: www.nimh.nih.gov/health/topics/anxiety-disorders/index.shtml.

174 Depression: What You Need To Know. Mental Health Information. National Institute of Mental Health. https://www.nimh.nih.gov/health/publications/depression-what-you-need-to-know/index.shtml.

175 Depression complications can affect many facets of your life. https://www.webmd.com/depression/guide/depression-complications#1.

176 Verhoeven, JE.et al. *Major depressive disorder and accelerated cellular aging: results from a large psychiatric cohort study.* Mol Psychiatry. 2014.19(8):895-901; Depression and Older Adults. National Institute on Aging. https://www.nia.nih.gov/health/depression-and-older-adults.

177 Burton, N. *Is Greed Good? The psychology and philosophy of greed.* Psychology Today. Oct 6, 2014.

178 Seltzer, LF. *Greed: The Ultimate Addiction-What's the unquenchable thirst for wealth all about*? Psychology Today. Oct 17, 2012.

INDEX

O

P

S

T

V

Made in the USA
Middletown, DE
25 September 2020